LOSING MY PATIENCE

WHY I QUIT THE MEDICAL GAME

Mickey Lebowitz, M.D.

>> North Syracuse, New York <<
<< Gegensatz Press >>
>> 2009 <<

362. 1
Lebowitz M

Cataloging-in-Publication:

Lebowitz, Mitchell Ross (Mickey), 1958-
    Losing my patience : why I quit the medical game / Mickey
Lebowitz, M.D.
        Includes bibliographical references.
        ISBN 978-1-933237-22-0 (e-book)
        ISBN 978-1-933237-26-8 (softcover)
1. Physicians—United States—Biography. 2. Physicians—United States—
Attitudes. 3. Health Care Reform—United States. 4. Medical Care—
United States. 5. Lebowitz, Mitchell Ross (Mickey), 1958- .
[DNLM: 1. Practice Management, Medical—economics. 2. Personal
Narratives. 3. Physicians. 4. United States. 5. Endocrinology. 6. Lebowitz,
Mitchell Ross (Mickey), 1958- . WZ 100 L436 2009]
I. Title.
        R154 L436 L436 2009   610/.92 B—dc22   AACR2
Library of Congress Control Number 2009926334

First edition. Printed in U.S.A. by United Book Press, Baltimore.

The guillemets, or two pairs of opposing chevrons, dark on the lower
cusps and light on the upper, are a trademark of Gegensatz Press.

Distributed to the trade worldwide by:
Gegensatz Press
108 Deborah Lane
North Syracuse, NY 13212-1931
<www.gegensatzpress.com>

Cover by Saairah.
Layout by Eric v.d. Luft.

Table of Contents

Prelude

Starting about 2002, I began writing down events on my office notepad pertaining to my practice of medicine. I chronicled what made me happy or sad, laugh or cry, want to sing or want to scream. I kept these scrap notes on my desk in steadily growing piles. I did not know why I felt compelled to write down these daily happenings, although catharsis quickly comes to mind. Over the ensuing years I noticed that I was writing more and more of the unpleasantness of being a physician, a sign to me that the aggravation level of practicing medicine was exceeding the satisfaction level. Then, in 2007, when I closed my practice, I felt the need to share my story, hoping that "putting a face on a problem" might serve to help others understand the plight of the modern American physician.

I am typically not a public or confrontational person, but, after significant scrutiny, I decided to use the notes to write this book. My reasons for doing so are three: First, writing it was a way for me to vent, which I felt was therapeutic, healthy, and less expensive than seeing a psychologist. Second, I felt that I owed my loyal and dedicated patients a thorough explanation of why I left them in their time of need. Maybe then the patients of other physicians who left their practices would understand why their physicians left them as well. Third, and maybe most important, I hope that my story, which I believe is shared by many physicians, may contribute to health care reform in the twenty-first century.

I wish to thank, in alphabetical order, Mustafa Awayda, Paul Cohen, Mark S. Erlebacher, Julie Fenster, Aaron Fey, Tim Green, Arlene S. Kanter, Steven Kepnes, Eric Luft, Bart Natoli, Susie Rosenwasser, Janice Scully, and Robert Weisenthal. Your help and contributions are truly appreciated.

I dedicate this book to my wife, Anne; my children, Rachel and Sam; my parents, Nat and Gloria Lebowitz; my in-laws, Lowell and Ruth Ruffer; my patients; and my colleagues.

Introduction

The Golden Years are Gone

For the first two thirds of the twentieth century any physician in America who was willing to train and work hard could put up a shingle and have a successful solo medical practice, close personal bonds with patients, and little outside interference from non-physicians. Moreover, such physicians could feel like they were making genuine and worthwhile contributions to the health of their communities. For some, these may have been the golden years of medicine. But the game changed in the last third of the twentieth century and the beginning of the twenty-first.

Insurance companies have assaulted physician autonomy in treating our patients and running our practices. They have usurped our medical and financial decision-making. This, without improving patient care, has skyrocketed the costs of keeping medical practices open and of health care in general. Pharmaceutical companies have taken luxurious profits, to the detriment of our patients, many of whom cannot afford our prescribed treatments. Lawyers and politicians have thwarted malpractice reform while some physicians' malpractice insurance premiums have increased beyond affordability. Malpractice attorneys, hiding behind their mask of protecting the patients, have typically accepted only those cases that would profit them the most. All this continues to happen as government officials sit idle, with lobby money from special interest groups pouring into their coffers.

Such intrusions into our practice of medicine have left many physicians angry, frustrated, and so disillusioned that many have considered leaving their practice, and others, like me, have actually done so. This is my story.

Code A

"Code A!" blared across the hospital's loudspeakers. "Code A, sixth floor!" the operator's voice echoed again at full volume. It was 1986, in the wee hours of the morning of one of my first nights on call as a second-year resident physician. I had been working nonstop since 7:00 the morning before. Exhausted and bleary-eyed while admitting my umpteenth patient from the emergency room (ER), "Code A!" made my eyelids pop open, my heart rate quicken, and my spine shiver. "Code A" meant that someone was suffering a cardiac arrest. I was the one responsible for saving that person's life. Game on!

I yelled to my intern and medical students, "Let's go!" We started running to the elevator but I said, "No time, take the stairs!" We hoofed up the six flights, two steps at a time. Out of breath, sweat dripping off of my face, and my heart jumping out of my chest, we arrived at the patient's room where he lay in his bed attended by a respiratory therapist, who was forcing oxygen into his lungs through a mask, and a nurse, who was doing chest compressions, counting with each push "one, two, three, four, five ..." Then all eyes focused on me. Trying to look calm, even though my insides were revving to my own adrenaline, I received a quick briefing about the patient. He was a thirty-six-year-old male who had recently received a heart transplant, but it was failing.

I had pictured this scene in my mind so many times in the past and had practiced it endlessly in controlled laboratory settings, but now it was for real. "How are you going to handle it, Doctor?" I said to myself.

"Paddles please for a quick look," I said to the nurse. Placing the paddles on the patient's exposed, motionless chest, I immediately recognized that he was in ventricular fibrillation ("v-fib"), a lethal heart rhythm if not treated immediately. "Prepare to defibrillate at 300 joules." As soon as the defibrillator was charged, I yelled, "All clear!" and delivered the electricity. His body jumped but remained flaccid. I saw no response on the heart monitor, still "v-fib." Without hesitation I ordered, "Charge to the max, 360!" and just as quickly I delivered the second shock.

"C'mon, c'mon!" I silently prayed to myself. "Convert, convert! Come back, come back!" Then it happened. I heard music to my ears, a regular beeping from the heart monitor, a sign that the heart had restarted. I glanced quickly at the monitor. It showed a normal heart rhythm. I was exhilarated and relieved at the same moment. "Check for a pulse." "Present," replied the nurse who was doing the compressions." "Check for a blood pressure." "Present," replied my intern. "Yes!" I reflected to myself, "Life saved!"

Although deep down I wanted to do an end zone dance like football players do after scoring a touchdown, instead, pretending I had done this before, I nonchalantly thanked everyone for their efforts, put a note in the chart giving the details of the event, and went back to the ER to continue my shift of thirty-plus hours. But all I could think about as I slowly walked down the six flights was how I loved being a doctor.

But times have changed. Almost twenty years later, it was my clinical practice and medical career that was in "v-fib." In fact, as I write this in early 2009, the entire U.S. health care system is in "v-fib." Was there anyone to deliver the shocks to save me and my practice? Is there anyone to save the system at large? Sadly, the answer, so far, has been no.

I Threw in the Towel, but I'm Still in the Game

Now I know what Hall of Fame basketball coach Bobby Knight must feel after a referee makes an unfair call against his team: like throwing a chair and cursing. I can easily relate to his anger, frustration, and distress. When I was in undergraduate school, I considered studying political science or criminal justice with the idea of going to law school. In the end, however, I decided against that plan because I imagined practicing law would be too adversarial for my personality. I am inherently a lover, not a fighter. I wanted to be in a career where it was all for one and one for all, where there was no greed or self-interest. Where we would all lock arms, work together, and sing "Kumbaya."

I dreamed that the practice of medicine would fit those criteria. It would be extremely challenging but worth the enormous personal sacrifices. I imagined it would not be adversarial. I pictured that everyone involved, the patients, doctors, pharmaceutical and insurance companies, and the policy makers, would work together, "united we stand, divided we fall," toward one goal only: the health of our patients. I was wrong.

In 1978 I was twenty years old, playing point guard for the State University of New York (SUNY) Oswego basketball team. The other team was bigger, stronger, and faster. "What we have to do to win this game is stop them from running, jumping, shooting, and hollering," my coach urged during his pre-game pep talk. Despite his fervent directives and our team's determination to fight bitterly to the end, we were soundly defeated. My teammates and I were upset that we lost, but we knew the season was not over yet. We looked forward to our next game.

I hated losing, and now, thirty years later, I still hate losing. The rival now is a group I will call the "other team." This team's players consist of insurance companies, pharmaceutical industries, and government officials. Ready to come off the bench at any time are malpractice attorneys. Unlike my time on the SUNY Oswego team, I have been playing against this team for a long time — over sixteen years. But just like that game in 1978, beating them has been impossible. I have thrown in the white towel. After sixteen years, I left my general endocrinology practice on October 31, 2007.

I considered moving on with my life and leaving behind my medical community, thousands of patients, my hard-earned reputation, and the prestige that was still associated with being a clinician. I thought I could accept that I was just another casualty of the contemporary health care system. I planned that I would find another job, any job, as long as I could earn enough to pay my bills and I would no longer be playing against the "other team." I would try not to have any bitter feelings, pretend not to care about the injustices done to me and my patients, and not take it personally. I played and lost. That is how games go.

However, my conscience will not let me just move on and I cannot pretend that I do not care. I have too much of a commitment to "my team," i.e., my patients and my colleagues, to just toss the ball aside and walk away. Like my teammates, I have invested too much time and energy studying, training, and honing my skills to leave my beloved profession behind without a fight. I have seen too many injustices for me to stay silent. Although I have stopped working as a practicing endocrinologist, I feel compelled to speak up for my team in hope that the American medical system will change.

My story, my team's story, needs to be told. Physician dissatisfaction is increasing as the "other team" jumps higher and faster. The best, most dedicated physicians are frustrated from their constant defeat against the forces of the insurance and pharmaceutical companies and the malpractice system. This is a critical time in American health care. If the "other team" truly believed that patients and not profits matter most, and if their ego, greed, and self-interest were locked up forever, then we could have a great game where everybody would win.

This book is a true and honest account of my journey from my undergraduate years through medical student through practicing physician and my struggles with the "other team" all along the way. In it you will find my questions, struggles, and stories of my patients. It also contains research on the problems in the American health care system in the early twenty-first century, as well as reflections on the state of physician morale and the shortage of primary care doctors. I wrote it from , the depths of my heart and soul and from the point of view of a physician who has been in the game, seeing patients all day every day while trying to survive the health care system. It is an urgent cry for change in our health care system and the polices that govern it. With the writing of this book, I hope to call the "other team" on all their fouls — and even some of my own team's fouls.

Chapter One

This is My Story: Good News / Bad News

There was no other way to say it to my wife. Just a year earlier, on October 31, 2006, I had blurted out, "I have good news and bad news. The bad news is, they are closing my practice. The good news is, they are closing my practice."

She knew that "they" were my employers. I will call them "Family Physicians of America (FPA)." They were like most primary care physicians in America, working long hours and seeing increasing numbers of patients each day in order to offset their ever rising expenses — all this at a time when reimbursements from insurance companies and Medicare were stagnant or declining. Before I joined FPA in 2004, it was looking for creative ways to enhance its revenue. I already knew many of the partners from medical school and was comfortable with their medical and business skills. We formulated a detailed business plan based on accountings from my previous practice.

In 2004, when my negotiations with FPA began, I was a physician in a clinical diabetes and endocrine practice owned by one of our local hospitals. Like the doctors in FPA, I was seeing more patients and working longer hours than ever before. Because I had no other endocrinologist with whom to share coverage after office hours, I was on call 24/7. I was wearing out and needed to make a change. My hope was that joining FPA would give me the ideal place to treat my patients. After one other change of practice, from fee-for-service practice to hospital practice in 1998, I was optimistic that this would be the last time I would ever have to move.

Our goals of combining our practices were clear. First, I would continue to take excellent care of my endocrine patients, especially those afflicted with diabetes. We had hopes and expectations of improved reimbursement from the insurance companies. Second, FPA agreed to expand its pharmaceutical-sponsored clinical research program. This was a win-win program for everyone. The patients would receive free medicines and examinations and the pharmaceutical companies would have their medications accurately studied. It would be intellectually satisfying for the physicians to study new medications and it had the potential to turn a profit. Our third goal was to attract new endocrinologists to our community; this would also enhance our first and second goals.

My practice was to be a subdivision of FPA called the Diabetes and Endocrine Center (DEC). As their employee, I would receive a guaranteed salary for practicing medicine. They would manage the business of the practice. These were the financial rules of the game: If the revenues of my subdivision exceeded its expenses, they would keep the overflow; if the revenues were less than the expenses, they would make up the shortfall. I accepted these rules and played this game to the best of my ability.

I Just Wanted to Be a Physician, Not a Businessman

My basketball coach used to scold me when I tried to do something beyond my abilities. "Mickey," he would shout, "do what you do best." As an employed physician, I felt I could concentrate solely on what I do best: treating my patients. My salary would be stable from year to year. I could also eliminate any potential conflict of financial interest related to either treating patients or ordering tests. I had already sold all my pharmaceutically connected stocks in an effort to remove any outside influences on my decisions regarding patients. More than ever, I could now focus solely on what would be best for my patients.

From Fee-for-Service to Employed Physician

The idea of becoming an employed physician had first appealed to me after having been in a fee-for-service private medical practice from 1991 to 1998. During that time, each year I worked longer hours and saw more patients. Yet, because of the insurance companies' policy of reducing our reimbursements and our ever-increasing office expenses, our incomes decreased each year. I tried to see more patients each day, even if that meant spending less time with each one. This was not good for the patients or for me. I certainly did not go into the practice of medicine to "rush 'em in and rush 'em out." I was deeply concerned with the quality and safety of patient care. Despite my deep affection and admiration for the physicians in that group, I left it for a situation that I expected to be better for my patients and for me.

I became an employed physician in 1998, working for one of our local hospitals in downtown Syracuse. I was the founder and medical director of its DEC. My office was across the street from the hospital and connected to it via an underground tunnel. Although this was convenient for me to juggle my very busy office and hospital practices, especially during our snowy winters, it was inconvenient for many of my patients to travel downtown and even more inconvenient for them to park in the large, confusing parking garage. They grumbled about paying for the parking too, especially if I was late seeing them for their appointments, because the meter was running.

Most significantly for me, I was on call all day every day, as there were no other endocrinologists with whom I could share coverage. In addition to long daytime hours in the office, I was in the hospital mornings, nights, and weekends. Whenever I was out of town, I took my cell phone with me, at least, to be available for phone consultations. I was suffering from battle fatigue. Moreover, I always felt guilty: Either I did not have enough time to spend with my family or I was unable to keep up with reading the current medical literature. Eventually I limited my priorities to family, my own health, and my patients — in that order. I gave up nearly all my outside interests. No longer did I serve on my children's school board or coach their sports teams. I stopped attending sporting and cultural events, and even limited my time spent socializing. I missed countless out-of-town family events due to lack of time or energy. Normally a happy and positive person, trying always to see the world as a "half-full" glass, I was becoming negative. I was not "me." I did not want to continue living like this.

My Story: The End

I was optimistic in 2004 that moving my practice from the hospital to FPA would allow me to make constructive changes in my life. We would try to recruit more endocrinologists to reduce my patient load and, perhaps most importantly to me, as a matter of my own well-being, I would not have to see patients in the hospital. I notified my patients that I was eliminating my hospital practice. I planned to be home every night with my wife and children. The hospital doctors, hospitalists, would care for my patients who were admitted after I gave up my hospital practice. Although perhaps not optimal for patients and their continuity of care, this arrangement was becoming more popular among doctors because it did not require them to go to the hospital, made their office practices more cost-effective and efficient, and allowed them still to have personal lives. The business part of my practice would be managed by an expert businessperson. On paper, at least, it looked like the perfect game plan.

Our plan was successful in providing excellent, conveniently located medical care. We expanded the DEC to include an additional endocrinologist and a nurse practitioner. We began doing clinical research. But soon the practice began to fail financially. Despite the fact that I saw more patients and generated more revenue than ever before in my sixteen-year medical career, the DEC lost money each month, which was understandably intolerable for FPA. Based on 2004 data from the Medical Group Management Association (MGMA), I generated more revenue than most endocrinologists, putting me in one of the highest percentiles. But this was not enough. The DEC had to close. It could not survive in its current medical marketplace

So, just like my basketball team back in 1978, my new

team and I, despite having a good game plan and playing our hearts out, lost to a much bigger and stronger opponent. This time, however, our rival was the "other team" — the insurance and pharmaceutical companies, the malpractice system, and the government. In the end, FPA decided to close its DEC for business reasons. FPA sent a letter to my patients, informing them that my practice would be closing in five months, on October 31, 2007.

Treating Sugar is Not Financially Sweet — Prevention Does Not Pay the Bills

We were not the only diabetes practice to become a financial casualty. In 1999, Beth Israel Medical Center in Manhattan and three other well regarded New York City medical institutions started diabetes centers to maximize treatment for New Yorkers, who were developing diabetes at an exponential rate. But within ten months of opening, Beth Israel had lost 1.1 million dollars. By 2006, three of the four centers had closed, despite the doubling of the incidence of diabetes in New York City. Their doors closed, not because they could not serve the medical needs of their patients, but because they could not sustain their programs financially.

Well known in the medical/financial world is that the way to make significant money in medicine is by treating the complications of a disease, not by preventing those complications. People who suffer from diabetes, for example, may require regular foot exams by a podiatrist. As perverse as it sounds, some insurers may refuse to pay $100 or so for each such preventive foot exam, but, as Ian Urbina pointed out in the January 11, 2006, *New York Times*, they would be willing to pay $30,000 for an amputation! Ironically, Urbina's article was called "Bad Blood: In the Treatment of Diabetes, Success Often Does Not Pay."

In the 1990s, a colleague and I developed a diabetes education center for our entire community to help people afflicted with diabetes to learn how to manage their conditions.

As an endocrinologist, I was one of his advisors. Highly skilled nurse educators and dieticians gave instruction and information on diet, exercise, medications, how to check blood sugars, the significance of blood sugar readings, and the goals of therapy. We measured the success of our program, and found that after only a few months our patients' blood sugar levels were significantly better. Lower blood sugars correlate with fewer and milder diabetic complications. Despite the patient benefits of the program, it hemorrhaged money and closed within one year.

Over the previous ten years, I could count approximately eighteen local providers who had treated diabetes and endocrine disorders and who had died, retired, or left their practices. Some were casualties of the contemporary health care system. Given the nationwide paucity of endocrinologists, very few replacements are available in the first decade of the twenty-first century, leaving many people with diabetes and other endocrine conditions without adequate specialty care.

I Did Not Think it was Fair to be Penalized

I could have remained at the DEC, but that would have required many changes to my philosophy and practice of patient care. I would have had to see more patients each day, for less time each, just like I did in my first practice, risking both the quality of patient care and my own well-being. "Been there, done that." This was unacceptable to my patients and to me. Alternatively, I could work the same hours and at the same rate but take a substantial salary cut. Work faster, harder, longer, or be financially penalized? Neither choice was agreeable to me.

I did not want to spend less time with my patients. I was the coach and they were my players. Adequate time with them was crucial to providing them with the quality of care to which they were entitled. For me quality of care means treating their complicated conditions, such as thyroid disease and diabetes, educating them about their conditions, and, perhaps most importantly, developing their trust. We were a team. I gave the instructions but they had to carry out the play. They would not be able to manage their conditions on their home courts outside the office without learning the appropriate skills at my office and believing in my advice.

Over the years, I constantly modified the way I took care of my patients, understanding that all I had to offer them were my skills and service. My goal was to hear them say, "That was the best medical experience I ever had." To accomplish this goal, I revamped my office hours. The first consultation with a new patient was always an hour, but instead of scheduling subsequent office visits for ten or fifteen minutes, I scheduled them for twenty. In this way my patients did not feel rushed and, most of the time, neither did I. As a result of the longer office visits, I typically ran only fifteen to thirty minutes late, instead of my previous thirty to sixty-minute delay. This improvement was an acceptable amount of time for most patients. Since I no longer had hospital hours, my office hours ran from 7:30 a.m. to 4:00 p.m. instead of 9:00 a.m. to 3:00 p.m. The extra office time was better for my patients and me as well.

Most of my patients were very happy with the care they received from me and my staff. I suspect that if an exit poll had been taken, our approval rating would have placed us high in the standings. I think I had many more wins than losses. Most important to me, however, was that many of my patients left the office better than when they came in.

I never thought I was doing anything special in the way I treated my patients. My coach used to tell me, "Do the basic things right." I did. I treated every patient the same way I would want my family or myself to be treated. I set up the exam room so that we all faced each other; sat and listened to their concerns before I asked questions and did my exam; gave them information and recommendations in words that they could easily understand; and, given my dreadful penmanship, had my nurses write out instructions for them if necessary. There are only two people in the world who can read my handwriting, and I am not one of them.

All my patients were star players, regardless of race,

religion, gender, size, shape, or social status. I treated a U.S.
ambassador, a factory worker, a teacher, or a person without
insurance all with the same respect, kindness, caring, and
competence. When it all came down, they each had similar
fears and concerns and shared the overriding desire to be well
and feel well without pain or suffering.

Although I merely treated patients the way I was taught
to do in medical school, the patients' response to my care was
humbling. At times their gifts, kind comments, and letters of
gratitude overwhelmed me. Every year since 1996, I was ho-
nored by my colleagues selecting me to be on the *Best Doctors*
lists for either Central New York, the Northeast, or America.
I must have been selected for these prestigious lists for doing
something right. Therefore I had no desire or motivation to
change my style of practice. Specifically, I did not want to
spend less time with my patients. Although I felt that the system was mistreating my teammates and me, I would not in
turn mistreat my patients. So what was the alternative? To
take a significant pay cut? I would not do that either.

I did not pursue a career in medicine to make a lot of
money. My motivations were much more idealistic than that.
Like most physicians, I wanted to help the world, even if it
was only one person at a time. However, I did not think it
was fair to be financially penalized when I, my patients, and
my colleagues believed that I delivered excellent care to my
patients. The problem really was not the reduced amount of
money itself. I could still stay in practice and earn enough
money to satisfy me and my family even with a salary cut. It
was the principle that offended me the most.

Did Anyone on the "Other Team" Care that the Practice was Closing?

In the end, I did consider taking a salary reduction so that I
could remain in practice and serve my patients. I dreamed,
however, that it would have to be under one condition: that
the insurance companies' CEOs and executives would take a

salary cut as well. All for one and one for all, right? How could I justify making less money when each year they were making more or, in fact, taking more? For example, William W. McGuire, M.D., CEO of UnitedHealth Group from 1992 to 2006, made 124 million dollars in 2006 alone, which did not include his hundreds of million of dollars in shady stock options; and when he resigned effective December 1, 2006, amid a securities scandal and the threat of federal prosecution, his golden parachute was approximately 1.1 *billion* dollars. Such crooks are the stars of the "other team."

If an insurance company had a financial shortfall, it could raise patient premiums or reduce my reimbursement for an office visit. If I had a financial shortfall, I could either increase my patient load per day, cut back my own expenses (even though we were at bare bones already), or take home less pay. Furthermore, I was the one on the front line, delivering the day-to-day care to the patients, seeing them in the office, and taking their phone calls at night. I was the one with the full responsibility and potential liability. I believe that my approval rating was much higher than that of the insurance companies' CEOs. Yet, despite all that, I dreamed that if they had ever been even remotely willing to take less money, I would have done so as well.

My business manager contacted representatives of the largest insurance carrier in our area, Excellus Blue Cross / Blue Shield, to tell them that our DEC was closing for "business reasons." We could not financially sustain the practice with the reimbursements we were receiving. Representatives of that company responded, "We will take this under advisement." *Under advisement?* Did that mean that they did not care? How could they not care? There was a shortage of endocrinologists and an epidemic of people with diabetes. Were they not concerned that there would not be enough specialists to see their insureds? Were they not concerned with the increased future risks and costs of acute and chronic diabetic complications?

I was cynical, suspicious that, because of the nature of the people I treated, Excellus Blue Cross / Blue Shield was secretly happy that we were closing. These patients had advanced medical problems that required several medications and multiple tests. These medications and tests are expensive and require insurance payouts. Maybe they hoped that if a non-endocrine specialist, who would be so overburdened with so many other patients and paperwork, were treating these complex patients, then that other physician would not have the time or knowledge to order all the tests and medications that I knew to order. Thus, without these tests and meds, their insurance payouts would be less, and they would keep more money for themselves. In the end, and rather quickly, their profits would increase. Maybe this insurance company assumed that some of these patients would leave their insurance plan in the near future, and that their medical issues would thus become another insurance company's financial problem. I believe that this is the mindset of the insurance companies, putting quarterly profits above the long-term health of their clients.

Before we closed our practice, my nurse practitioner contacted our state and local government officials to see if they could somehow put pressure on the insurance companies to improve their reimbursements and thus save our DEC. She received no reply from our state officials. Perhaps they were too busy to respond. Maybe they did not understand the problem. Or — and I hate to think of it — could it be that they just did not care? Could they have been more beholden to insurance industry lobbyists than to the citizens who had elected them? Nor did she receive any replies from our local politicians, with the exception of one state senator, who is also a medical malpractice plaintiff's attorney. Consider the apparent conflict of interest. In my more cynical moments I even thought that maybe he wanted us to stay in practice because eventually, he believed, we would make a mistake and he could sue us. In the end, my nurse practitioner met once with one of his assistants, but we never received any follow-up from that visit.

No Last-Second Victory

When my patients were notified of my practice closing, there was a significant uproar. People were very upset. Their unhappiness with the situation was palpable. Phone calls came into my office from angry, frustrated, and disappointed patients. They were looking for someone to blame. "Who put you in this situation," they exclaimed, "the government, insurance companies, FPA?" Patients sent strong letters protesting our closing to me, the owners of the practice, and the local newspaper. There was an article in the paper and even a short segment on one of our local TV news shows about our decision to close.

Although I did not necessarily intend my decision to leave medical practice to be a catalyst for change, it was exciting to speculate that maybe there were unseen benefits to my leaving. Perhaps a grass roots movement was forming to change the system. Who else besides the patients could possibly push the "other team" to change the health care system? I imagined them revolting with a good old-fashioned march on City Hall or maybe even the White House. Maybe something positive would really happen. Maybe there was a silver lining. I walked around my house humming the Buffalo Springfield song, "For What It's Worth."

But the emotions and energies soon fizzled out. There were no follow-up articles in the paper, no more TV stories, and no more angry letters or phone calls from my patients. I do not think that this was because people stopped caring. Certainly it was not because anything improved. I suspect that people were busy just trying to live their own lives or that they became overwhelmed trying to find other doctors. In short, life went on. There are only so many times that doctors or patients can be knocked down running into the line of the wealthy and powerful "other team" before they realize that they are getting nowhere. I believe that this is the "other team's" plan, to wear us down, like Muhammad Ali's "rope a dope" plan for the "Rumble in the Jungle" in 1974 and the "Thrilla in Manila" in 1975, when he just rested on the ropes of the boxing ring, taking punch after punch after punch, round after round, until he wore down both George Foreman and Joe Frazier, then went on the attack and defeated them.

In the end, there would be no fourth quarter comebacks, no one coming out of the bullpen, to save the DEC. It was over.

I Gave the Fist Sign

In college, when we became exhausted during a basketball game, our coach had instructed us to raise our fist, give him "the fist sign." He would then take us out of the game and give us a rest. FPA was only asking me to leave its practice, but I was certainly free to continue to practice medicine, just somewhere else. I was then in a situation to make what I anticipated to be a very personal and potentially life-changing decision.

Thankfully I had options: many offers to join other established medical groups. But as I explained to my wife, the bad news was that, if I wanted to stay in practice, it would be more of the same. Like many other full-time private practitioners, I would continue with the long hours, the financial stresses, and the risks of litigation, as well as the negative intrusions on patient care by insurance and pharmaceutical companies and the government. Prospects looked bleak. Maybe this was the time to give the fist sign and escape from this unfair game.

The good news was that this could be an opportunity to leave the practice of medicine, even though I believed that I was then at my professional peak. Like many other physicians, I felt too fed up, cynical, and angry with the health care system, and too used by the "other team" to make their exorbitant profits, to be able to continue with my principles under constant attack. I could use the closing of the DEC as an excuse to my patients, colleagues, friends, and family, and leave semigracefully.

I would no longer need my daily pep talk, "You can do this. You are strong. Today will be better. Just give it your best. Do it for the patients. Do it for the team." I would not have to psych myself up with each step during the morning routine that got me closer to answering the bell so that when I walked through the office door I would be ready to play.

In the end, I decided to give the fist sign. I lost my

patience with the system and left my patients. That broke my heart. For now, my clinical game is over. I admit that the "other team" can run, jump, shoot, and holler better than I can. Though I may be sitting on the sidelines, I have not quit my team. I still want to play, but from a different position. I am hopeful that I can still help my team to win by giving voice, our voice, to improve the health care system.

Chapter Two

Studies and Stories: I Am Not Alone

My feelings are not unique. Like many physicians, I have frequent opportunities to talk with other doctors at medical society meetings, national educational seminars, or local educational lectures and round table discussions. I cannot remember a time when physician morale was so low and the whining, complaining, frustration, and anger levels were so high.

Physicians' negative attitudes toward the American health care system in the first decade of the twenty-first century remind me of the story of Sodom and Gomorrah in Genesis 18:16-19:29. God told Abraham that He would destroy Sodom because it was so full of sin. Abraham negotiated with God and God agreed that, if Abraham could find fifty righteous people there, then God would spare the city. A short time later, Abraham came back and said to God, how about forty-five righteous people? Then a short time later, he said to God, how about forty? Then, how about thirty? Twenty? Abraham finally argued God down to ten righteous people but God would go no further. In the end Abraham could find only one righteous person, Lot, so God destroyed the city, and Gomorrah as well, but saved Lot and his two daughters. The analogy is that I am pessimistic that I could find even one physician, never mind ten, twenty, thirty, forty, forty-five, or fifty, who is totally satisfied with this health care system and all the parties involved in it. Maybe the whole thing should be destroyed with fire and brimstone.

Doctors are being trampled by a system that we are desperately trying to survive. We feel beat up, worn out, and many of us are burned out. Many persist stoically onward and upward, moved by devotion and obligation to our patients. Some stay for financial reasons. But so many doctors are unhappy with their careers. Alcohol and drug abuse rates are disproportionately higher in doctors than in the general population, as are suicide rates, especially among women physicians.

Married physicians also suffer higher divorce rates than the general population. Even I, someone who tries to appreciate life's wonders and live every moment to its fullest, have had dark thoughts. We are the ones responsible for our patients' good emotional and physical health, even as we ignore or lose our own.

"Job Satisfaction in the United States," a survey published on April 17, 2007, by the National Opinion Research Center (NORC) at the University of Chicago, concluded that, despite our incomes and social status, physicians scored lower (fifty-eight per cent) than physician assistants (seventy-eight per cent) and clergy (eighty-seven per cent) did on measures of job satisfaction and did not even make the top twelve on the list. On September 24, 2007, LocumTenens.com reported on its Web site <www.locumtenens.com/physician-careers/Business-of-Medicine.aspx> that ninety-seven per cent of 2400 surveyed physicians felt frustrated by the non-clinical aspects of their profession. These aspects include insurance and Medicare reimbursement problems; medical liability concerns; federal regulations, policies, and procedures; and administrative and business agendas. These all interfere with clinical decision-making and impinge directly on the quality of patient care. The long work hours, probably due at least in part to the aforementioned issues, were a major problem too. According to Merritt, Hawkins, and Associates, a national recruiting firm, new physicians and specialists are moving toward employment positions with the relative security of a weekly paycheck instead of opting for the significant challenges of operating solo or small group practice businesses.

Contrast these 2007 studies with data from the 1990s. In the November 19, 1998, issue of the *New England Journal of Medicine* (*NEJM*), Dr. Jerome P. Kassirer wrote an editorial entitled "Doctor Discontent." Using surveys that measured the level of dissatisfaction, he described the frustrations that physicians experienced. He quoted a 1995 survey that found forty per cent of 1700 physicians spending less time with their patients compared with three years prior and sixty per cent having serious issues with the external forces on their individual practices of medicine. At that time, "only" thirty-three per cent of physicians were either dissatisfied or very dissatisfied with their practice of medicine.

The March 2005 issue of *Physician's Money Digest* (*PMD*) reported on three surveys. The first, in 2001, found that seventy-five per cent of physicians in California were less satisfied practicing medicine than they had been five years earlier. In the second, a 2003 Kaiser Family Foundation survey, eighty-seven per cent of queried physicians stated that the morale of their colleagues had declined, and sixty per cent felt that their own morale was lower compared with previous years. The third, done in 2003 by Merritt, Hawkins, and Associates, showed that after only two years in residency, twenty-six per cent of medical residents would not have chosen a career in medicine again if given the choice.

In 2007, a survey of 1200 physicians by the American College of Physician Executives (ACPE) found two out of three doctors felt emotionally burned out and six out of ten had considered leaving the practice of medicine. What would happen to health care in this country if six out of ten physicians actually followed through and left their practices?

These studies confirm my anecdotes, conversations, suspicions, and deep concern that many more physicians like me will leave their practices also. Who then will take care of the patients? Will insurance company CEOs and executives with their excessive salaries come to the medical office after we have left and treat our patients, ill with diabetes, hypertension (high blood pressure), hyperlipidemia (high cholesterol), or vascular disease? Will they send their financial officers and vice presidents to deal with Addison's disease or Hashimoto's thyroiditis?

Dr. C.

A bittersweet article appeared in our local newspaper in 2008 about a physician whom I will call Dr. C., who reluctantly left his rural practice after twenty-five years of dedicated service.

He worked long hours in the office and even made house calls when needed. An icon in his small town, Dr. C. barely made it financially. He took whatever the insurance paid when the patients were covered by insurance and he did the best he could for those with no insurance. Due to his intense commitment and loyalty to the locals, he remained in the community, essentially working for almost no pay, until he could find a suitable replacement to take over his practice. It took five years for Dr. C. to find a physician he could trust with his patients. During those last five years, he took on extra work and hours outside his practice, working as a part-time hospitalist and organizing a family practice residency program, so that he could financially support his own family.

Dr. C. grudgingly gave up his fight with the health care system when he left his community practice. He then went to work full-time as a salaried employee, taking care of sick patients in the hospital instead of trying to prevent illness and keep people out of the hospital.

I know Dr. C. personally. He is a "doctor's doctor," a person anyone would want to have as her/his physician. He is dedicated, smart, kind, easy to talk with, and non-judgmental. Although Dr. C. is special, he is not unique. Many internists and family practitioners have given up the hassles of clinical practice and the goal of disease prevention. Instead, they have chosen to join hospitals as salaried, employed physicians with regular, predictable hours and without the aggravations of operating small businesses and being beholden to insurance companies and to Medicare's reimbursement whims.

The Looming Primary Care Shortage

From 1980 to 2000, the U.S. population grew by twenty-four per cent, from 226 million to 281 million. Between 1960 and 1970, two doctors graduated from medical school for each doctor who retired. At the beginning of the twenty-first century, only one new doctor enters the field for every one that leaves. At that rate, by 2015, it is projected that new doctors entering the field will be fewer than those doctors retiring from the field.

In 2009, many physicians are considering leaving their practices, but the proportion of students applying to American medical schools is, at best, flat. There are just over two students vying for every available medical school position in the U.S., compared to four for every spot in Canada. One major reason for this difference, according to Gail Morrison's "Mortgaging Our Future: The Cost of Medical Education" in the January 13, 2005, NEJM, may be the high price of medical school tuition and fees. This price can be as much as $50,000-$60,000 per year for private American medical schools, which is sixty per cent more than for comparable Canadian institutions. This article noted that various governments fund medical schools in many countries outside the U.S. Morrison's article also stated that sixty per cent of all American medical students grew up in the wealthiest one fifth of all American families. This suggests that middle and working-class Americans are underrepresented in the profession. Despite these gigantic costs to attend medical school, the American Association of Medical Schools (AAMC) has proposed increasing the number of future medical school openings by 3000, thus raising the number of medical school graduates each year from 16,000 to 19,000.

Some leaders in the field, however, do not believe that the correct prescription for alleviating the looming shortage of primary care providers is to increase either the number of medical students or the funding for these institutions. David C. Goodman and Elliott S. Fisher wrote in their April 17, 2008, NEJM editorial, "Physician Workforce Crisis? Wrong Diagnosis, Wrong Prescription," that, rather than spend more money on funding medical education, we should reallocate existing money toward primary care, geriatric, and prevention fellowship programs, in addition to expediting reform of our contemporary reimbursement system.

As of February 2009, there were no plans to increase the number of residency positions, which total about 24,000 openings per year. The number of new doctor graduates from American residency programs will likely remain close to constant. This situation makes less opportunity for foreign medical graduates to enter American residency programs. In 2004, 215,576 doctors were international medical graduates (IMGs), making up 25.6 per cent of physicians practicing in the U.S. At that time, these IMGs were more likely to practice internal medicine than other specialties, as Elie Akl, Reem Mustafa, *et al.*, reported in the February 2007 issue of the *Journal of General Internal Medicine.*

This comes at a time when the need for medical care is expected to grow, as our baby boomers age and as our citizens become more obese, with all the attendant medical consequences. Although there are more doctors per capita in 2009 than ever before, there are projections of a physician shortage, especially in primary care. In "2005 Physician Supply," in the November 2005 installment of *Hospitals and Health Networks* online magazine at <www.hhnmag.com>, Dagmara Scalise suggested that the shortage might be as many as 200,000 by 2020. This trend is already a reality, with rural populations being the main victims. In 1970, primary care physicians, whom researchers found to value interpersonal relationships, independence, and public service over wealth or prestige, made up 40.2 per cent of the total number of doctors, with the remainder of physicians practicing in specialty fields. By 1980, the percentage of primary care doctors had dropped to 36.5 per cent, and by 2004, 33.5 per cent.

This disparity between primary care providers and specialists might become even worse as the costs of medical education grow, leaving more medical school graduates with higher debts. They would then need to pursue the higher paying, procedure-oriented specialty fields, rather than primary care. Only one out of twenty-two residents graduating in 2009 from the SUNY Upstate Medical University internal medicine program plans to enter the field of primary care. The remainder will pursue specialty fellowships or employed hospitalist positions. (Many of these residents are IMGs, whom we used to expect to go into primary care.) When queried informally about their desire not to pursue careers in primary care, the repeated theme of their answers was that primary care physicians do all the scut work that nobody else wants to do, and are undervalued and underpaid compared with specialists, despite their intense commitment to patients. This shortage of primary care physicians, and even endocrinologists, could be exacerbated by physicians, like me, leaving their practices prematurely, at the peak of their game. It does not even take into account the tsunami of uninsured patients without primary care doctors. These patients will be looking for doctors if the health care system ever changes and requires everyone to have a primary care provider.

It appears that the days of doctors practicing into their sixties and seventies are gone. According to American Medical Association (AMA) statistics reported by Wendy Abdo and Mike Broxterman in the June 2004 *Physician's News Digest (PND)*, thirty-eight per cent of the 884,974 physicians in the U.S. were over fifty while only 162,364 were over sixty-five. The AMA and Merritt, Hawkins each consistently find that a full eighty per cent of physicians over fifty consider retirement from full-time clinical practice during their next five years. Their decisions are based, at least in part, on their concerns about the insurance and governmental policies that are discussed in this book. Furthermore, doctors are more often choosing employment instead of self-employment, and employed physicians are likely to retire earlier than their self-employed colleagues. This trend will also reduce the physician workforce. Also, the 2007 Retention Survey of the American Medical Group Association (AMGA) and Cejka Search found that the number of physicians choosing to work part-time increased from thirteen per cent in 2005 to nineteen per cent in 2007. The greatest numbers of part-timers are aged thirty-five to thirty-nine. This trend toward part-time was seen in both men and women.

According to the Doctors Company, the nation's largest physician-owned malpractice insurance company, sixty-six per cent of physicians would dissuade their children from entering what I still think is one of the noblest and most potentially satisfying of all professions. This sad fact contrasts to a generation ago, when two thirds of surveyed doctors encouraged their children toward pursuing careers in medicine. The 2006 movie, *Blood Diamond*, highlighted this concept. In the film, the father, Solomon Vandy, dreamed that his son would survive the horrible atrocities and savagery occurring in Sierra Leone at that time, become a doctor, and do good for the world. But when I asked my usually loquacious daughter if she wanted to be a doctor, she gave me a succinct, uncomplicated response, "Hell No!" In response to the same question, my son just looked at me in silence, incredulous that I would even ask him anything so absurd. They had witnessed how their old man worked. They had heard first-hand my grumblings about the "other team" and saw the effects it had on me, including the long hours and the stressful days and nights, and the accelerated balding and graying. They wanted no part of it.

Across the country, as many as one out of five physicians no longer practice clinical medicine. They are either retired, doing research, administration, or something unrelated to medicine — all kinds of things except treating patients. This totals approximately 180,000 doctors in the U.S., who could help to care for our citizens, but for some reason are choosing not to do so.

I know several local physicians, men and women alike, who continue to face significant challenges trying to balance their work and family lives. Many of them feel as though they are on the junior varsity team, because they choose to work part-time in order to spend more time with their children. They feel that the varsity players, the full-timers whose main priorities are their practices, do not respect them. This negative attitude appears to be changing, at least in the Netherlands. According to Marjolein Lugtenberg, Phil Heiligers, *et al.*, in "Internal Medicine Specialists' Attitudes Towards Working Part-Time: A Comparison Between 1996 and 2004," in *BMC Health Services Research*, October 2006, full-time internists regarded their part-time internist colleagues "slightly" more positively over those eight years. Even if this attitude becomes more positive in the U.S., it will, in combination with our baby boomers aging and our senior physicians leaving, likely exacerbate the looming primary care shortage unless we fix our health care system — soon.

Chapter Three

The Years in Training

I must confess that I thought about leaving medical practice as far back as my first few years in practice in the early 1990s. Even then, it was easy to see that being successful in the business of medicine was not as simple as hanging up a shingle and watching the patients and the money roll in. On the contrary, physicians' decisions regarding patient care were already being usurped by Medicare and insurance companies' guidelines — not to mention the persistent concern that any mistake or unexpected negative outcome might incur a lawsuit.

I feel guilty that I had such thoughts, because one of the happiest days of my life was when my father screamed to me over the phone in April 1981, "Mickey, are you sitting down? Are you sitting down? You got in! You got in!" I started at SUNY Upstate Medical University that fall and graduated four years later, in 1985. Going to medical school, however, unlike for some, for me was not a lifelong dream. In fact, while growing up, the thought of a career in medicine was never even in the ballpark.

Play Hard but Play Fair

I grew up in a working-class neighborhood in the Canarsie section of Brooklyn. My middle-income parents were loving and hard-working. I had a younger brother and an older sister. Several of my aunts, uncles, cousins, and grandparents lived in close proximity. Picture a Neil Simon play — that was us. None of my grandparents, aunts, uncles, or parents graduated from college. They were all bright, intelligent people who, unfortunately, did not have the time or money for college. They had to go to work to make money to survive.

In the streets of Brooklyn, which my parents called "the gutter," I played punchball, stickball, spongeball, stoopball, and handball. My friends and I were not great athletes but we played each game as if it was the national championship and we always played fair. When we divided the teams, we always tried to make them even. We knew, even as kids, that it was wrong to give one team a sizeable advantage over the other. This is the way I imagined it would be when I grew up: play hard, play fair, and keep both sides equal.

As a youth, I was an extremely intense and competitive player. This desire to play my hardest and win persisted when I played basketball in college. I had nicknames like "The Spark" and "Tasmanian Devil." At the end of each practice or game, I would be exhausted, literally crawling to the locker room. That is how I played basketball and that is how I practiced medicine. Sometimes at the end of a typical office day, I felt that I needed someone to pick me up and take me home, and I only lived eight miles away! None of my patients ever suffered from a lack of effort on my part.

Though I never dreamed about becoming a doctor as a child, I now realize that, like many physicians, I had many of the personality traits necessary to be a physician, such as determination, focus, altruism, idealism, fierce competitiveness, and being the supreme team player. Although I relish winning, I value fairness and equality more. This belief has made it very difficult for me to exist happily in a medical world where the sides are not equal and the teams are not fair for either the physicians or the patients. My high expectations of what a medical career was supposed to be made my eventual fall from my dreams to medicine's reality even harder.

I Found My Way in the Holy Land

The idea of becoming a physician first occurred to me while studying at the Hebrew University in Jerusalem during my junior year of college. For the first time in my life, intensely goal-oriented students from the Ivy League and other highly prestigious colleges surrounded me. These students were bright, motivated, and had professional aspirations like law and medicine, but certainly did not walk on water. I realized that I could play in their league and have the same aspirations that they did.

I was originally attracted to the healing profession because of pain that I suffered as a senior in high school. I broke my foot and missed almost the entire basketball season. Because I was the type of person who lived to experience the most each day, being injured was a serious setback for me. I believed that if there was anything I could do to help others from feeling the way I did, then I was willing.

Before I went to Israel, my plan was to become a physical therapist, combining that field with my love of sports. But after my experiences in Jerusalem, I decided to go to medical school. I gave up my volunteer position at the school for the deaf in Jerusalem — I was then also considering a career in special education — as well as any notion of being a sportscaster or disc jockey, which had been the original reason I went to college. I volunteered at Hadassah Hospital in Jerusalem.

Living in Israel was my first personal experience of intense hatred and disdain displayed by one group of people against another. For terrorists, life was cheap. The more people they killed, the better. I did not envision the world this way. To me, life was precious. The way the body functioned was magical. How could anyone try to destroy any human being just because of different skin color or religious or political views? I was desperate to find a way to make the world better.

When I returned to the U.S., I began working in a nursing home as a nurse's aide in order to test my desire to pursue a career in medicine. I wanted to make sure, before I committed to the enormous amounts of time, energy, and money that it would take to become a doctor, that I felt comfortable around frail people with advanced illnesses. To see other sides of the medical life, I also volunteered in emergency rooms, radiology offices, and microbiology labs. When I saw men and women suffering, I found myself drawn to them. This feeling reassured me that my decision to go to medical school was right. I knew that I could not save the world as a medical doctor, but I hoped and dreamed that I could make it just a little bit better.

If You Tell Me I Can't,
It Only Makes Me Try Harder

For me, the road to medical school had major obstacles. Although I thoroughly enjoyed my first two years at SUNY Oswego — maybe too much at times — I thought that I would have a better chance of being accepted into medical school from an institution that is well known for its premedical program. I applied to transfer to Cornell University but was rejected. OUCH! I was never really rejected before, except by a few women who were probably out of my league anyway. Instead of pushing me to quit, this rejection only increased my desire to persevere. So I returned to Oswego and was promptly rebuffed by the premed advisor. Given the relative scarcity of premedical students and successful medical school applicants over the years, his position at Oswego was rather lonely. I still do not know if his tactic was reverse psychology or if he was just being realistic. All I know is that if anyone ever tells me that I cannot achieve something, it only increases my resolve to achieve it. I transferred my competitiveness and determination from the basketball court to the classroom. In fact, my favorite inspirational poem, written anonymously, is:

If you think you are beaten, you are. If you think you dare not, you don't.
If you'd like to win, but think you can't, it's almost a cinch you won't.
If you think you'll lose, you're lost. For out in the world we find
Success begins with a fellow's will. It's all in the state of mind.
Life's battles don't always go to the stronger or faster man
But sooner or later the man who wins is the one who thinks he can.

Because I had decided on medicine in my senior year, I needed to spend a fifth undergraduate year at SUNY Oswego to complete the prerequisite classes for medical school. To expedite my application to medical school, I audited an organic chemistry course during the summer, while working in a nursing home. I also studied for the Medical College Admission Test (MCAT) and took the test the following fall. At graduation, having finally earned my degree in zoology, I received both the Zoology Student of the Year and Student Athlete of the

Year awards. I now had the credentials to gain acceptance into medical school: a high overall grade point average, an excellent average in my core zoology courses, decent MCAT scores, and many extracurricular activities. Moreover, it did not hurt my application at all that one of the other players on my college basketball team was the son of the Dean of Admissions at the SUNY Upstate Medical University College of Medicine. As you may imagine, I (intentionally?) passed the ball to his son a lot.

My college basketball coach used to say to all of us, "It's only fun when you win." When I was accepted into medical school, it was as if I had won the national championship, but the "fun" was just beginning.

Hard Work and Long Hours? Sign Me Up

Medical school at SUNY Upstate Medical University was, as one may imagine, difficult, but oddly enjoyable. No more was I learning for the sake of good grades. Instead, I would actually need to use the information that they taught us in class. One studies very hard if someday a person's life may depend on what one knows. We were constantly tested by written and oral exams. The amount of information we were required to learn and retain was, at times, overwhelming. Just when I felt like there was no more room in my brain for any additional information, they gave me more to study and yet another test. Rigorous? An understatement. I still cannot believe I did it.

While in medical school, I knew that being a physician was going to be physically and emotionally demanding. Long hours and intense content would get to us. I also realized that we would often experience difficult situations where our ethics, morals, and values would face challenges. I realized that we might feel isolated or afraid to show any signs of weakness when discussing difficult real-life issues. How would we deal with cancer patients who refuse treatment, preferring to go "naturally," or with patients' spouses who contract sexually transmitted diseases from extramarital affairs? What would we do for patients with serious side effects from medications we had prescribed, or who suffered because we missed the diagnosis? How would we cope with the profound grief of losing our patients to death or with the anxieties of having to make life-or-death decisions? Would we stay silent and suck it up? Would we become depressed and irritable? Would we turn to alcohol or drugs? Would we feel like killing ourselves? How could we become comfortable talking about these difficult issues? I chose to do what I do best. I initiated a group called "Students Supporting Students," a formal opportunity for open discussion of different opinions on handling these intense, challenging situations. Many medical schools have since installed actual curriculum to help medical students understand and deal with these complicated issues.

I did well academically, frequently making the Dean's List and the Medical School Honor Society. I studied diligently, in part because I felt that I had something to prove to my naysayers. In pursuit of my desire to make the world better, I volunteered for various medical school committees and was awarded the Community Service Award after my second year of medical school. At graduation, with my parents, in-laws, and many of my aunts and uncles in attendance, I received the Stuart I. Gurman, M.D. Award, "given to that graduate of high scholastic achievement who best showed a continuous interest and activity in art, music, literature, or the public interest, realizing that living and learning go together."

I Am Glad I Did It but
I Never Want to Do It Again

After medical school, I stayed in Syracuse to do my internship and residency training at SUNY Upstate Medical University. I fell in love with Syracuse when I came south from Oswego every Friday night on the bus, an hour each way, to volunteer in the University Hospital ER. Syracuse is a curious mix of a blue-collar town and a college town. It has a great sports tradition, lakes, mountains, and room to move — very different from growing up in metropolitan New York. It is a friendly, affordable place to raise a family. In 1985 the hassle factor was low, the convenience factor was high, and getting from place to place was easy. As Syracuse was relatively traffic-free, if I needed to drive somewhere in ten minutes, I could comfortably leave nine minutes and fifty-nine seconds before and still be on time. I used this time tactic almost every morning during residency, trying to squeeze in every last bit of sleep and still be on time at the hospital. My "time neurosis" about efficiency, trying to be well-organized so I could have some free time, a technique that I would later need while attempting to stay effective in private practice, started during my internship. Our senior residents would frequently admonish us, "Only touch the paper once!" and "Work quickly but do not rush!" Difficult tricks indeed.

During training, the only thing that was even remotely glamorous about being a doctor was being able to call myself one. Internship and residency were exactly as advertised. The hours were incredibly long, and every third day we stayed overnight in the hospital, working as long as thirty-six hours. Some weeks I worked 120 grueling hours. We used to joke with each other about our machismo and that being on call "only" every third day made us miss two thirds of the cases, as we were not in the hospital the other two nights. But the hours were no laughing matter. If I was not working, studying, in the bathroom (where I would sometimes study to save time), being embarrassed by one of the senior attending physicians for not knowing the answer to some trivial question, or stressing about whether I had given the correct treatment to my patient, then I was sleeping. It was insanity, sold to us as a way to get optimal medical experience. Or maybe it was a rite of passage that was passed down through the generations in order to become members of the medical establishment. We all knew that, if nothing else, we provided cheap labor for the hospitals. Our salaries, considered in relation to hours worked, were less than minimum wage.

One Person Can Make a Difference

In 1988, one year after my residency finished, the Bell Commission enacted the Libby Zion Law. She was the eighteen-year-old daughter of Sidney Zion, a lawyer and columnist for the *New York Daily News*. She died in 1984 at New York Hospital in Manhattan, at least in part because of a missed diagnosis. It was alleged that first and second-year medical residents mismanaged her care. These residents were suspected to be, at least in part, sleep-deprived, overworked, and responsible for upwards of forty other patients in the hospital. Studies have shown, and I can validate, that sleep deprivation impairs one's judgment and ability to make sound decisions. Thanks to Sidney Zion, who relentlessly campaigned for regulations to restrict medical residents' hours, residents since 1988 have been limited to no more than twenty-four hours in a shift and no more than eighty hours in a week, and must have at least one day off each week. The Institute of Medicine (IOM) has further restricted residents' hours, so that, as of 2009, a resident may work only sixteen hours maximum without sleep, must have at least ten hours off between shifts, and must obey limits on moonlighting. Moreover, the IOM limits the number of patients that a resident may admit and care for at one time. Many studies in the *Journal of the American Medical Association* (*JAMA*), *NEJM*, and other important medical publications have all consistently shown that longer hours lead to more — and more serious — medical errors.

Sadly, although many of us acted strong and tough, the hours were, and still are, emotionally draining. A summary of studies on this topic, published in *Annals of Internal Medicine*, March 5, 2002, looked at internal medicine residents working the reduced eighty-hour work week. The findings showed the burnout rate for these residents to be over seventy-five per cent. This meant that three out of four residents who were not even in practice yet — where, I can attest, the work and stress are much tougher — were already exhibiting symptoms of burnout. This research found that "burned-out residents were more likely to say that they discharged patients early to make their work manageable, did not fully discuss treatment options or answer a patient's questions, or made medical errors" (p. I29). More than half were unhappy to have chosen medicine as a career while twenty-five per cent stated that, given the choice of career, they would not select medicine again. Burnout may be defined as emotional exhaustion, depersonalization, a feeling of low accomplishment, a high rate of cynicism, decreased or suboptimal job performance, and just going through the motions without passion, interest, or commitment.

According to the AAMC 2006 Graduation Questionnaire, eighty-seven per cent of new medical residents were in debt, owing a median amount of $130,000. A full fourteen per cent had debt levels above $200,000. The average income for medical residents, after eight years of education, was between $40,000 and $50,000 per year, or about $12 per hour for an eighty-hour work week. Some had little disposable income, especially if they lived in large, expensive cities and needed cars to drive to the different hospitals that they had to cover. Some could not even afford safe housing. Given these financial challenges, and in spite of their already long hours, some residents had to take part-time jobs just to make ends meet, especially if they had families to support. Thus it was no surprise that more than one of three residents exhibited symptoms of depression while six of ten were cynical about their medical training.

Details Really Matter

Internship and residency were times when I discovered that details mattered. Small errors in judgment, lack of knowledge, or poor communication with other staff or patients could lead to significant patient injury and even death, as well as litigation. I will never forget the elderly man, suffering from chronic alcoholism, who voluntarily came into our Veterans Administration (VA) hospital for a safe detoxification. Unfortunately, he developed significant alcohol withdrawal symptoms, for which we gave him Valium around the clock. While in the intensive care unit (ICU), he vomited and aspirated his gastric secretions into his lungs. At the time, despite our specific orders that the head of his bed should be kept constantly elevated, a seemingly small detail, he was lying flat in bed. He went into cardiac arrest requiring resuscitation. Even though he survived, he suffered hypoxic encephalopathy (lack of oxygen to the brain) and was never the same again. Witnessing the consequences and ramifications of such errors helped to shape the way that I practiced medicine when I entered clinical practice. I became compulsive about details, which frankly was not a trait that I had had prior to my medical training. Paradoxically, the longer I practiced medicine, the more time it took me to see each patient, because, now that I knew what to look for, I did not want to miss any important details.

I performed well as an intern and resident and was given the William Schiess Award for the medical resident who best personified Dr. Schiess's outstanding characteristics of service, leadership, and loyalty to the highest ideals of the profession of medicine. Dr. Schiess was an leading internist in our community and one of the founding fathers of one of Syracuse's most reputable internal medicine practices. Along with two of my closest friends from training, I was also rewarded with an honors year to be one of three chief residents. Our responsibilities were to teach the newer residents, organize and oversee educational conferences, and help to untangle tough house staff problems. It was also a year without overnight call. I admit that I really needed and wanted that chief year, to recuperate from the sleep deprivation that I had incurred during the previous three years.

Chapter Four

Endocrinology

"Are You Sure You Want to Be an Endocrinologist? You'll Have to Take Care of Diabetes"

During my chief year, I decided to specialize in endocrinology, diabetes, and metabolism. Endocrinologists diagnose and treat glandular diseases. Sometimes this is confused with "swollen glands," which commonly occur when people have viruses and other infectious diseases. Those "swollen glands" are really lymph nodes, an important part of the body's defense system. Unlike endocrine glands, lymph nodes do not secrete hormones. By definition, endocrine glands release their hormones into the blood stream where the hormones have effects on the body in other locations.

There are many hormone secreting glands. These include the pituitary, called the "master gland" because it controls several other endocrine glands, such as the thyroid at the base of the neck in the front, the two adrenal glands that sit like hats on top of each kidney, and the sex glands, the ovaries in a woman and the testicles in a man. The pituitary also produces the milk hormone, prolactin, so that women can nurse their babies, and the growth hormone that allows children to grow into adults.

There are other less well known endocrine glands: The four parathyroids, located behind the thyroid, help to regulate calcium levels in our bodies. C-cells, located within the thyroid, produce a hormone called calcitonin which can have an impact on our bone densities. The gastrointestinal tract produces a variety of incretin hormones, the most notable being GLP-1, secreted from the terminal part of the small bowel, the ileum. The level of GLP-1 is important in the management of type 2 diabetes. The pancreas, located behind the stomach and in front of the spine, produces many different endocrine hormones, most notably insulin, produced from its beta cells.

I chose endocrinology because the professors were Jedi masters, the science was spectacular, and the patients' problems were incredibly challenging. Having never even dreamed when I was a child of being a physician, here I was becoming an endocrinologist. In fact, there may be only one child in the history of the world who said when he was young that he wanted to be an endocrinologist, and that is my son Sam. When his sixth-grade teacher asked the students in his class what they wanted to be when they grew up, many chose teacher, firefighter, or police officer, but Sam's response was unusual. He stated that he planned to become not only a doctor, but an endocrinologist! This was before he understood what it took to go to medical school and survive postgraduate training and clinical practice.

Each field of medicine has within its discipline medical conditions that some physicians may find less appealing to treat. For example, I considered being a gastroenterologist, but I would have had to deal with stool samples and perform colonoscopies. Colonoscopy procedures were, and still are, financially rewarding. To a gastroenterologist going into the rectum with the scope is like entering a gold mine; but to me it is still just a rectum.

As it turned out, nothing could have been more exciting over the years than seeing the progress made in understanding all aspects of diabetes mellitus. In fact, my favorite saying in this regard has been, "If you ever had to have diabetes, now is the time to have it," because each year its causes are better understood and its treatments are more effective than the year before. Those who do not have diabetes may easily take for granted their body's ability to use the food that they eat. They may not realize that, independent of what or how much they eat, whether they are extremely active or not, whether they are emotionally or physically stressed or not, their body will produce the exact amount of insulin that they each need. This is a miracle indeed!

What I also loved about treating endocrine diseases in general, and diabetes in particular, was that it forced me to learn in intricate detail all the body's organ systems. Diabetes potentially affects the eyes, kidneys, nerves, and vascular system. In addition, it is frequently associated with high blood pressure and cholesterol problems, two common conditions that pose treatment challenges. Both can increase the risk of vascular disease, heart attacks, and strokes, the leading causes of death in people with diabetes. Moreover, any acute medical condition, physical or emotional, could adversely affect a diabetic's blood sugars. Hence treating people with diabetes also required me to care for the body and the mind together. In that way I inadvertently became a practitioner of holistic medicine. I came to understand the difficulty of coping with, and the challenges of living with, a chronic condition. Having a chronic condition is like having a prison sentence, only there is no time off, even for good behavior.

Every day in the office, at least one patient with diabetes would literally cry about this dreaded disease. Patients were concerned with fluctuating blood sugars, or upset about taking numerous pills and needing insulin injections. It takes incredible discipline and motivation for an individual to treat or manage her/his own diabetes. I came to believe that, before anyone could be afflicted with diabetes, s/he should have to pass a test. Passing the test would prove that a person was ultra-smart, dedicated, ambitious, motivated, emotionally stable, and able to deal with unexpected situations. Only those who passed would be allowed to have diabetes. Unfortunately, there is no such test and, as we were told in kindergarten, in life, you get what you get.

In the end, I was not only a diabetologist, but also a behavioral therapist and a quasi-psychiatrist. In fact, the most interesting aspect of being this kind of physician was not so much knowing and treating the disease process itself, but witnessing my patients' emotional responses to their medical conditions. To deliver optimal medical care to my patients, I had to be flexible, constantly adjusting my approach to each individual based upon their different needs. My motto was certainly *not* "my way or the highway" and one size surely did not fit all.

Chapter Five

The Practice Years

It Was Downhill from There

I was thirty-three when I got my first real job, starting practice in 1991 with a large multi-specialty group. I had finished five years of undergraduate studies, four years of medical school, three years of training, one year as chief resident and two years of endocrinology fellowship, a total of fifteen years of schooling. Thankfully, I was in only moderate debt because I went to public undergraduate and medical school. Thus I had the option to choose internal medicine and endocrinology, my true passion, instead of a higher-paying specialty that would have allowed me to pay off a larger debt.

Even early during my training years, I detested the hours and the loss of life's balance. I thought that this was a rite of passage, and that my life would improve once I got into practice. But when, over the years in practice, the situation only got worse, I tried to determine the source of the problem. Was it the specific situation in which I worked? Or, were there larger outside influences, such as the loss of autonomy, financial issues, threats of malpractice, or inherently endless hours, all made worse by the insurance companies' and Medicare's declining reimbursements associated with increasing practice expenses, that combined to make my job unsatisfying? Whatever the reason, it was becoming increasingly difficult for doctors like me, through little or no fault of our own, to help nice people like my patients.

I tried changing my practice from fee-for-service with the multi-specialty group to being an employed physician with the hospital in a small endocrine practice. I attempted to continue to treat my patients with diabetes and other unusual endocrinopathies for their internal medical conditions as well, acting as a holistic doctor, as suggested by our American College of Clinical Endocrinology (ACCE). When that became too time-consuming and financially challenging, I reluctantly eliminated those non-endocrine responsibilities from my practice and had the patients establish with separate primary care physicians for their non-endocrine conditions. This change in our relationship was painful for both my patients and me.

Because of the outside influences, throughout the years and in different practice settings, the aggravations often exceeded my satisfactions. I persevered, because I enjoyed treating my patients and receiving excellent feedback from them, and from my colleagues, that I was playing well, doing a good job. I was, in many respects, a victim of my own success. The better I took care of patients, the more patients were referred to my practice. As much as I may have wanted to, I could not duplicate or franchise myself like a McDonald's or an Arby's. The busier the practice, the longer my hours and the more I had to deal with the "other team." I did not want to change the behaviors that had made me successful, i.e., spending time with patients, listening to their concerns, and communicating my diagnosis and treatment plans to them in words that they were easily able to understand.

As a professional, I found it impossible to say no to my colleagues or friends who wanted me to see their patients, especially when my teammate physicians were playing just as hard as I was. Working part-time was not an option for me, because I did not feel that I could take care of my patients according to my standards with that type of schedule. Another reason for persisting was the amount of time, energy, and money that I had already invested to become a physician. How could I leave now? I was also concerned about my colleagues' opinions of me. I did not want them to think of me as weak or a loser, traits that an ultra-competitive, relatively young man like me could not tolerate. Then there were the patients to consider. Who would take care of them if I left, especially with the dearth of endocrinologists in our area?

Through the years in practice, I was extremely frustrated and angry about the inequities and injustices that I regularly faced as a physician. I would often ask myself whether I was unhappy with the practice of medicine. Perhaps those issues were really just within me. Perhaps I was depressed or anxious. However, I did not feel depressed, nor did I exhibit any of the usual signs of this condition. I did not feel burned out either. Up until my last days in practice, I gave my patients my maximal attention and effort.

My ninth-inning attempt to be content with the practice of medicine, to stay in the game as a clinician, to take optimal care of my patients, and to have a personal life came when I joined FPA. We did clinical research. There was no hospital call. My patients and staff were happier. There was free parking. Nevertheless, in the end, the finances took us down.

Chapter Six

Should I Leave?

Consternation

I used to have a recurrent dream — or nightmare — about leaving practice. I typically do not remember my dreams, but I remember this one. I dreamed that I was Nell Fenwick (a weak and defenseless doctor?) tied to a log by Snidely Whiplash (the insurance companies? the policy makers?) in the Dudley Do-Right cartoon. I was about to go through the buzz saw. I kept waiting for Dudley (the medical society? the surgeon general?) to save me, but he never came to my rescue. I actually envisioned myself starting to go through the buzz saw, being split in half, but woke up in a cold sweat before I was halved too far. How would you interpret that dream? Half of me wanted to stay in practice, but the other half wanted to leave it all behind?

In Judaism there is a holiday called Rosh Hashanah, the Jewish New Year, two days of intense introspection and self-reflection. It asks one to question, "Is my life on the right path?"

What I anticipated and what ultimately came true was that, for me, the concept of Rosh Hashanah was taken to a new level. The DEC would close exactly one year after I was given notification. Therefore, instead of two days of intense self-reflection, I would have twelve months, reviewing the pros and cons of going into solo practice, starting a "boutique" or "concierge" cash-only practice, joining another general medical or endocrinology group in town, considering offers to unite with a nephrology or cardiology group, or leaving the practice of medicine completely.

I felt like I was in the interrogation chair of a detective's office, with the bright light on me 24/7. The interrogator was one of my mentors — or tormentors? — from internship. I pictured him: straggly hair, bushy eyebrows, top button open, tie pulled down to mid-chest, round face, rotund body. He was speaking to me, slowly, deliberately, with his New York City accent: "It's 3:00 in the morning." Pause. "No one else is around to help you with your decision." Pause. "So, what are you going to do, Doctor?" Pause. "What are you going to do?" Really long pause.

What was I going to do? The decision to leave or stay in practice haunted me day and night. It was the first thing I thought about when I opened my eyes in the morning and the last thought I had before I went to sleep at night. During the day, when I was not distracted by my patients, I thought about it again.

All of us, at one time or another, have had to make major decisions. For me the big-league decisions were: Which college should I choose? That was like shooting a lay-up. I went to SUNY Oswego because my friends Jimmy and Gerry were going. I could play basketball for the team. As a state school, it was affordable.

Should I marry my girlfriend? That was like tipping in a putt. Although I was "only" twenty-three, I proposed to my beloved. I knew that I did not have to look any further for my soulmate. We have to know when we have gold. I certainly knew when I had mine.

Should I have kids? That was like catching a lazy fly ball in the outfield, "a can of corn." I had always dreamed of having both a daughter and a son, so, when I saw those little testicles and "hooter" on my second child, after having had my daughter first, life could not have gotten much better.

Should I go to medical school? That was like kicking a soccer ball into an open net. Being a doctor would be the ultimate personal challenge, my own climbing of Mt. Everest, but without the extreme cold or the need for supplemental oxygen. It would be my chance to help my little corner of the planet, hoping to make it better, especially when there is so much suffering in the world.

But — should I leave my practice of medicine??? This would be the most difficult decision that I would ever have to make.

In retrospect, I realize that I had been planning to leave

my practice for years. But I wondered whether the right time would ever come. Would there ever be a right time? Then reality struck.

There was yet another denial from the insurance company or yet another preauthorization to fill out. There was yet another newsletter from our county medical society saying that our state legislature had rejected tort reform and that malpractice premiums were going up again, in addition to a $50,000 malpractice surcharge. There was yet another article in the *New York Times* about the numbers of uninsured people increasing while insurance company executives were making more money than ever. There was yet another patient who came to the office apologizing for not being able to afford the prescribed medications. There was yet another day with endless paperwork and patient hours, to try to make up for our financial shortfall. There was yet another phone call waking me up in the middle of the night, from a patient who was "having a hard time sleeping."

I considered what I would do if I did not practice medicine. I often found solace reading the classifieds in national medical journals. As soon as I received each issue, I would turn to the back pages and read the classifieds first, even before I had read the scientific literature. I dreamed about doing another job, sometimes almost any job, especially after a hassle-laden day and a long night on call. I was looking for a position that would challenge me and could make a positive difference in the world. If it had nothing to do with either the practice of medicine or the health insurance industry, I read on. Sometimes I did not care whether the job had anything to do with any aspect of medicine at all. Some days, when I came into the office and saw the maintenance engineer cleaning the hallways, I wanted to grab his broom, give him my stethoscope, and say, "Here, take this and you do it today." Maybe most importantly, I was looking for a job that would allow some balance in my life.

In 1996, Jeff Van Gundy took his first professional basketball head coaching job with the New York Knicks. I recall an interviewer asking him, "What is the most difficult part of your job?" He replied, "It's always on my mind." He would be thinking about it, not only during games, but during practice, while eating, and even while sleeping. His job was all-consuming. I felt his pain. It was the same for me, albeit without the glamour and pageantry of being a head coach in the National Basketball Association. When I came to the office each morning, no one on a loudspeaker yelled, "And now entering his office, the one, the only, Dr. Mickey Lebowitz ..." I did not enter my office each morning striding through fake fog. There definitely were no fireworks before I started seeing patients each morning, nor girls dancing for my staff and me during timeouts between patient visits, nor cheerleaders chanting, "DEFENSIVE medicine, DEFENSIVE medicine."

When I was not in the office or the hospital, I thought about my patients. Are they OK? Did I make the right decisions for them? Are they responding to the therapy? Are they getting better? Are they getting worse? Sometimes I would just call them at their homes. "Mrs. Smith, this is Dr. Lebowitz." Mrs. Smith would respond, "Oh, hi Mickey. Thanks for calling me, but why are you calling, it's Sunday night? I feel so much better with the new medicine. You can stop worrying." I knew that such phone calls were usually more therapeutic for me than for them. During residency, worried about one patient or another, I would often call the floor nurses to make sure all was fine before I went to sleep that night.

Although I spoke with my wife, friends, and parents, no one but me could make the decision to leave. In the end, they all admonished me to do what I thought would make me happy, what was most right for me. The most difficult part was that I always put them, my patients, and my teammates first. That said, time was running out on the clock, the final decision needed to be made. Should I leave? YES!

Response to "The Departure"

When my decision to leave practice was made public in our relatively small city, it seemed to me, at the center of the uproar, like the shot heard around the world. It reminded me of the phone scene in the Broadway show, *Bye Bye Birdie*. The news spread quickly: "What's the story, morning glory? What's the word, hummingbird? Have you heard? Dr. Mick is packing it in ..."

Parents of my kids' friends and even my kids' doctors questioned my kids about my decision to leave practice. My wife's friends and colleagues in her law firm queried her about my decision. I really had not anticipated that there would be this much interest. After all, many M.D.s leave practice every day, for one reason or another. However, many of those M.D.s were moving away, or retiring at an appropriate age. I was leaving in my so-called prime, when only a limited number of endocrinologists remained available in our community to take over caring for the thousands of patients in my practice.

Any place I went, whether it was the synagogue, the grocery store, or the barbershop, people would stop me and question me about my plans. Why are you leaving? Are you ill? Are you moving from the area? Joining a pharmaceutical company? Going into research? Going into teaching? But no one asked if I was going to be a model, movie star, or professional basketball player. Go figure ...

What was most interesting to me was the response from my teammates, colleagues, fellow physicians. One physician was ticked off. He communicated through one of our mutual patients: "Why doesn't he stick it out like the rest of us?" That was certainly not a ringing endorsement of how great it was to be a doctor in 2007.

Another physician was incredibly gracious and wrote me a letter thanking me for the years of service to our community and our mutual patients.

The most common response, by far, from other physicians in our community was, "I'm envious. I have been thinking about leaving myself. How did you do it?"

I found these comments to be depressing, sobering revelations of the contemporary state of affairs in being a physician in the U.S. at the beginning of the twenty-first century.

Could I Leave? Preparation Was Key

There were five seconds left on the clock when the coach called time out. We were down by one point and had the ball for one last shot. The crowd was screaming and it was hard to hear the coach in the huddle. He took out his eraser board and started diagramming a play. He only had one minute. Quickly, he drew Xes and arrows telling us how to get the ball in bounds and where to go once we did. The horn sounded to resume play.

I came off a screen and received the inbounds pass. Four seconds left. I passed it to one of our forwards standing on the foul line. Three seconds left. The other guard rubbed his man off on a screen and cut to the basket, he was open. Two seconds left. Our forward saw him free and passed him the ball. One second left. As soon as the guard received the pass he shot it. Swish. Through the net. The final buzzer sounded. We won! The crowd went wild.

After the game I went into the coach's office. He was seated at his old metal desk, busy reviewing the game's stats, and eating a sandwich. Without lifting his head he motioned with his hand for me to take a seat in one of the two chairs in front of the desk. "Coach," I said, "there were only five seconds left on the clock, the crowd was screaming, I could hardly hear myself think, and you came up with that play. How did you do it?" He immediately stopped what he was reading, finished chewing his last bite of sandwich, picked up his head, and looked me right in the eyes. He said, "I had this planned for a long time."

My coach went on to tell me that he had imagined one day this situation would arise: down by one, little time left on the clock, and our ball. If it ever happened, he would be ready with a play. We thought the coach was a genius for conjuring up the play to win the game, but he was *really* a genius because he was prepared. He had had a plan all along. I did not tell the other guys.

I Had a Plan for a Long Time Too

I felt distressed that I wanted to leave the practice of medicine after having been in it for only a few years. Was it possible that, despite all the time I had spent investigating a career in medicine by volunteering in health care related areas before deciding to pursue the costs and rigors of medical school, and despite all the time and effort I had put into medical school and the training programs, I had made the wrong decision?

Prior to joining "my team," I did not take into account the "other team" that I would be playing against, the insurance companies, the policy makers, the malpractice attorneys, the pharmaceutical companies, or their influence on the practice of medicine. In medical school, I spent all my time trying to learn the massive amount of material required. In internship and residency, as a new physician, just to treat the patients, to survive the arduous hours, and to stay awake was challenging and stressful enough. I never then considered these other players in the game. Not until I went into practice did I learn that it was not just about the patients and me. There were many other players who, although invisible in the exam room, influenced my decisions and, in general, our practice of medicine.

I knew early that having this "other team" involved, thus losing our autonomy in our interactions with patients and losing control of our finances, was not going to be survivable. I felt that they were usurping our beloved profession and that they were unstoppable. While we were treating our patients, it appeared to me and my colleagues that they were calculating, tweaking, and optimizing their attack plan. To make matters worse, their goals were diametrically opposed to ours. For clinicians, people matter most; but for the insurance industry, it appeared, sadly, money matters most. As physicians, we were being pushed to practice the art of business instead of the art of medicine.

They push us, the "providers" (the twenty-first-century term for doctors and mid-levels, i.e., nurse practitioners and physician assistants), to practice medicine in ways that they never taught us in medical school or training. See more "clients" (the twenty-first-century code word for "patients," people in need of medical care) each day. Take less time with them. Do not sit down. Stand with your hand on the door ready to leave. Do not ask them if there is anything more you can do for them today, for they may say yes. Gamble, take short cuts, and hope you do not miss anything, lest a patient should suffer or sue you for malpractice.

These business people control our medical decision-making. They require precertifications for medical procedures and preauthorizations for tests. They limit our choices of the medications that we can prescribe, despite having no medical education or experience in practicing medicine. They have never treated a sick patient nor taken a middle-of-the-night phone call from a patient in despair. They never even see or examine a patient. Nonetheless, they have become deeply involved in the decisions that we make. How do they do it?

I pictured that one day I, like my coach, would be in a difficult situation where I would be forced to make a difficult decision, and therefore, I too needed a plan if the situation ever arose. I felt like that time was now. I felt pushed to leave my practice, having to work in a health care system that valued profits over people and where my patients and I were pawns in a perverse game. It was a system controlled by insurance companies with policies made by politicians. The hours were endless. My wife would ask when I would be home and I would tell her, "When the work is done." There was too little time and energy left over to enjoy life's pleasures. The stakes were high and the threat of being sued for malpractice was ever looming. This was not what I envisioned or signed up for when I decided to pursue a career in medicine. Practicing medicine now felt more like a punishment than a noble, satisfying career. My plan was not to win a game; mine was a plan to leave medicine. I started planning in the early 1990s.

My plan to leave medicine had to address both emotional and financial components. I also needed to take into account my family's feelings about my leaving practice, not to mention the views of my patients.

My Plan — The Emotional Component

I began planning the emotional component by obtaining a copy of *Leaving the Bedside: The Search for a Nonclinical Medical Career* by Maija Balagot, Mark Ingebretsen, and Suzanne Fraker, put out by the AMA in 1992 and revised in 1996. Within this booklet were stories from other physicians about their reasons for leaving clinical medicine. These stories described their disillusionment with medical practice, third-party interference, financial issues, and threats of litigation. Some left because of their own medical problems. Some left to pursue careers in administration, research, or teaching. Some just left the whole thing behind and went into fields completely unrelated to medicine.

There were sections in the booklet where you had to ask yourself what it would be like for you, your spouse, kids, and friends if you were not a practicing physician, perhaps with lower income and loss of prestige. You had to answer the questions honestly regarding self-worth, obligation, and commitment to the community and the patients.

Another section was "The Courage to Change." The booklet stated, "Doctors, who are trained on a diet of duty, obligation, high achievement, and dedication can feel enormous conflict when they realize that the career in which they invested twenty years is not bringing them happiness." For a physician to change careers "requires a willingness to let go of the whole notion of what you are and how you want the world to see you." For me, I always felt like I was just "Mickey," who happened also to be a doctor. In fact, when I was introduced at my lectures, I would always say that I was Anne's husband and Rachel's and Sam's dad first and practiced medicine on the side ("M.D." stands for "My Daddy"). It has always interested me how doctors are called "Doctor" when most other people are not called by their job, as "This is Carpenter Smith" or "This is Teacher Jones." How did that happen? Among the few other professions that routinely do this are the clergy, e.g., "Reverend Johnson," "Father Davis," "Rabbi Levy," "Deacon Brown," or "Bishop Green"; higher education, e.g., "Professor Watson" or "Dean Schwartz"; and politics, e.g., "Senator Claghorn," "Mayor Lindsay" or "President Obama."

But how could I, even with my family and I emotionally prepared for me to leave practice, consider doing anything else, especially given my financial obligations to my family? I had a long-term plan for that as well.

My Plan — The Financial Component

During this time, I started reading about and became enamored with the concept of "voluntary simplicity," where having less is more. My motto over the years became, "The less I have, the happier I am." I was greatly influenced by Vicki Robin's and Joe Dominguez's popular book, *Your Money or Your Life: 9 Steps to Transforming Your Relationship with Money and Achieving Financial Independence*, which helped me to understand better what I truly wanted from money and how so many of us have been willing to trade so much of our lives for it. They raised the question, "Is making a living more like making a dying? Are we killing ourselves — our health, relationships, our sense of joy and wonder — for our jobs?" They added that "beyond a certain minimum of comfort, money is not buying us the comfort we seek." I agree.

Several years ago, my wife and I renovated parts of our forty-year-old house. When the job was completed, I said to her, "I am no happier than I was before the changes." It was clear to me that money truly did not buy happiness. The renovations were not worth the hours, aggravation, or stress that I was dealing with on a daily basis at work. In fact, there were many wealthy patients in my practice who were very miserable for one reason or another. Many of them had imbalances between their work and non-work lives. But how does one achieve simplicity when there are significant financial obligations?

Having money was never a big issue to me. (How could it have been an issue when I did not have any?) Everyone's relationship with money is personal. I grew up with little, although we always had "enough" food, shelter, and clothing. Like every kid, I wanted things, and on any occasion when I got "something," I really appreciated it, because I knew that it was a financial stretch for my parents. They were two extremely loving, hard-working people — no one could ask for better parents — but they did not hit the financial jackpot.

I remember when I finally got my new Sting Ray bicycle that I had wanted "forever." I faked that I was sick and could not go to school so I could ride the bike that day in our one-car garage. That said, I never needed much and never really wanted much material "stuff." I always went to public schools, including high school, college, and medical school. I worked as many as three jobs during the summer to save for school and was able to get by with very little "stuff."

If I had to go anywhere while I was in college, I would bum a ride or hitchhike. I was one of those people standing on the side of the road with the cardboard sign and my "hebe-fro" hair. Thankfully, I am still alive today to tell my story. When I took my spring break vacation during my sophomore year, I drove to Daytona Beach, Florida, with my best friend in his father's wood-sided station wagon. We gave rides to three girls from our schools who were willing to pay for all the gas. My friend and I slept in different hotels each night, or, I should say, in different hotel parking lots. We could not afford a room. The back of his dad's wagon made tight but affordable sleeping quarters.

I did just fine without a lot of money. I did not yearn for it and certainly did not want it to dictate what I would do in life. I just needed "enough." I did not think of chasing money as the game of whoever dies with the most wins. I was trying desperately not to trade my life for it. Yet this became a major dilemma.

I was working extremely hard to earn money, but not in order to buy "stuff" that I did not want or need, such as the biggest house, a second house, a fancy car, or expensive clothes. It just was not that important to me. Having "stuff" would not help me achieve my goal of making the world a better place nor would it make me happier — although if I ever had made it big, I would have loved to be a philanthropist.

In many respects I was, without knowing it, a prototype of the Easterlin paradox. In 1974, a University of Pennsylvania economist named Richard A. Easterlin argued in his article, "Does Economic Growth Improve the Human Lot? Some Empirical Evidence" (in *Nations and Households in Economic Growth: Essays in Honor of Moses Abramovitz*, edited by Paul A. David and Melvin W. Reder), that economic growth does not lead to personal satisfaction beyond being able to afford the basic necessities of life. What I really wanted most from money was choice: to stay in medicine if I chose or to escape if I felt like the rules by which doctors had to play were too harsh or unfair. I read many books like *The Millionaire Next Door: The Surprising Secrets of America's Wealthy* by Thomas J. Stanley and William D. Danko. I also began a very disciplined savings and investment program, following models like "dollar cost averaging" (DCA), diversification, and the "pay myself first" mentality. Before I bought any material "stuff," I would ask myself whether I really needed it, was it really worth my money or my life? I was not an ascetic, but I was careful.

My wife and I lived well but spent less income than we earned — she was working part-time as an attorney — and saved the rest. If any unexpected money arrived, we did not blow it; we saved it in what I called our "Escape Fund."

In the end, my response to the question of how I could leave my practice was, to quote my coach, "I had this planned for a long time." I would use the plan if the time were ever right. The DEC was closing for "business reasons." Our opponents were too powerful and could not be beaten. I felt that the rules of the game were lopsided and unfair. Our opponents must have figured that I would keep playing by their rules, because of my altruism and financial needs and obligations. They must have thought they had me beaten. But I had a plan and, again like my coach, the time came and the plan worked.

Chapter Seven

Would I Leave?

My ideals were very high. They have fallen a long way. My dreams of how things were supposed to be having turned into a nightmare, I feel like my altruism has been sucker punched. Each day I was in practice, I felt that in addition to putting on my white coat and grabbing my stethoscope to treat my patients, I had to put on my helmet, mouth guard, and cup ready to defend myself against the insurance companies, government policies, and malpractice attorneys. I also felt like I was always the visitor, playing on their turf with their rules and their referees.

Who Else You Got?

I did not think that leaving the patients would be as hard as it was. I used to say to my wife, "If I keeled over one day, and all my patients were there in front of me, sort of like in the Verizon commercial, they would, in unison take one large giant step over me. They would look down at me and in the same breath say, 'He *was* a good guy. Who else do you have to take care of me?' "

Some Were Angry

As it turned out, the outpouring of emotion from my patients toward my leaving was greater than I had anticipated. Many of their comments tested my decision to leave. Some were angry. For example, Stacy C. was a thirty-something-year-old, heavyset, hirsute female with type 2 diabetes, hypertension, and hyperlipidemia whom I had known for over ten years. After she received "the letter" she blurted, "Where the hell are you going? Who will take care of me?" I had treated her polycystic ovarian syndrome with metformin and she was able to conceive her one and only child. During her pregnancy, I treated the gestational diabetes she developed. I was also her primary care physician and treated her recurrent urinary tract infections (UTIs), gastro-esophageal reflux disease (GERD), and her profound iron deficiency. When she had marital discord, I counseled her and treated her depression. I knew her, her husband, and her daughter, who accompanied her to most of her office visits, extremely well. I understood her anger. I could not blame her for feeling that way.

Others were equally angry, though they expressed it differently. C.M., was a very pleasant middle-aged woman with advanced type 1 diabetes on an insulin pump. She also had kidney failure but was fortunate enough to have recently received a kidney transplant. C.M., whom I had known for several years, summarized her feelings in just two words, "This blows!"

P.C. was even more succinct. She was a cantankerous older woman who had been referred to my practice for management of her out-of-control type 2 diabetes. She needed insulin, but initially refused "the needle." We bickered back and forth like an old married couple, but I could tell that she was softening. At the end of our conversations she would laugh. She became nicer to my staff. I was gaining her trust, a key component in the treatment of diabetes. She finally acquiesced and started insulin. I told her that I would not let her walk through the forest alone with her diabetes and her insulin injections. I spoke with her by phone several times each week to optimize her insulin doses. She was feeling much better. She was jovial on the phone and in the office. She shed her crustiness. Before long, she allowed me to adjust her blood pressure and cholesterol medications as well. When she came to the office after receiving "the letter" that the practice was closing, P.C., the short talker, summarized her feelings in just one word, "SHIT!"

Not So Angry That I Was Leaving

J.C. was in her early twenties. She was being treated for hypo-thyroidism after having received radioactive iodine several years prior to treat her Graves's hyperthyroidism, mercifully without the bulging eyes. She was doing well on a stable dose of thyroid hormone. I only saw her once a year to check her blood test and renew her prescription. As I came into the exam room, she appeared to be sobbing uncontrollably, "boo hoo hoo," and rubbing her eyes. As I started apologizing for leaving the practice and began telling my, by now, well-rehearsed story, she stopped rubbing her eyes and said with a childish grin, "Gotcha!"

Similarly, Mr. P., an eighty-year-old man whom I was treating for a toxic multinodular goiter, waited in the exam room for an unusually long period the last day I was to see him. He said to me, slightly annoyed yet smiling at the same time, "This is the last time you'll keep me waiting this long."

I am thankful that no patient came into the office and said, "I am really glad you are closing your practice. I never really liked you and you never really helped me anyway."

I Felt Guilty Like Never Before

Other comments hurt me and raised my guilt to unprecedented levels — and that is saying a lot, as I grew up in a Jewish home.

"You're quitting? What a waste! What a shame. Where will we go for care? There are hardly any endocrinologists left in town." These comments were frequently echoed during the days, weeks, and months leading up until my last day in practice.

Mrs. M. laid into me as well. She was a thin, seventy-plus-ish woman whom I had known for years, treating her for diabetes with two shots of insulin each day. She had a raspy voice and spoke in the short phrases that are associated with chronic shortness of breath from years of cigarette smoking. She said to me, "You're too young (breath) to retire (breath).

How old are you (breath) anyway? Fifty-five?" She must have been reacting to my balding head, almost totally gray hair, and worn-out, haggard appearance. I said, "Mrs. M., I am only forty-nine. How old do you have to be to stop working?" "Well, at least (breath) sixty-five, or until I'm gone."

I reviewed the issues, telling her how the practice was losing money each month and how I could neither work any harder nor continue to compromise my principles. She was a frequent caller at night and knew first-hand how my hours were endless. I told her that I would be willing to make less money, but not while the insurance companies were taking more each year by paying us less and still raising the patients' premiums. She understood completely. Her husband had just passed away and she was having a hard time making ends meet, having to decide between food and medicine. Thank goodness she had stopped smoking. She confessed that she was in the "donut hole" — i.e., the coverage gap that she called the "loophole" — of her Medicare Part D and could not afford all her medications.

She admitted to taking her blood pressure and cholesterol medications only two or three times per week. She had stopped checking her blood sugars, because she could not afford the chemstrips for her glucometer — a very dangerous thing not to do, because she was now living alone and did not always feel her low blood sugars accurately enough to treat them. Untreated low blood sugars could result in insulin shock and possibly death.

My conversation with Mrs. M was repeated countless times each day with other patients. I rehashed why I was leaving and what the issues were. However, not all the conversations were painful. In fact, some were even comical.

Some Patients Felt Guilty

Some patients felt guilty themselves that I was leaving medicine. They thought it was their fault. L.W., a middle-aged attorney whom I had known for years, had had type 1 diabetes since childhood, yet he hated to have his blood drawn. Imagine the dilemma, a diabetic, requiring insulin, who hated needles. He was able to give himself insulin injections only because, thankfully, the needles were now sharper, finer, and smaller than ever, and it had become nearly painless to administer the insulin. Nonetheless, he would not let me take periodic blood samples to measure his kidney function, cholesterol, or blood counts, as recommended by the American Diabetes Association (ADA). He thought that I was leaving practice because he gave me such a hard time about drawing his blood. I reassured him that the issues were larger than that.

I had come across such needlephobia one other time with another diabetic patient. He had renal failure and was heading toward dialysis. I had to take blood samples to measure his body's chemistries if he was to remain alive. On one occasion, after at first having agreed to the venipuncture, he went ballistic on my phlebotomist when she tried to draw his blood. I suggested to him, later, after he had cooled down and apologized for his outburst, that he have a port placed to draw blood, just like people do who have cancer and need chemotherapy. (This is an example of the "art of medicine," using creativity and savvy to serve the patients best, that is usually not taught in medical school.) He agreed to the port and, although he still required dialysis, chose peritoneal dialysis instead of hemodialysis, because the former does not require needles. Managing his diabetes, cholesterol, and blood pressure then became much easier.

G.D., an African American woman in her late seventies, also felt guilty and responsible for me leaving practice. She was always pleasant when she came to the office, accompanied by her daughter. But, in spite of her advanced and poorly controlled diabetes, blood pressure, and cholesterol problems, she just would not follow my instructions regarding her treatments. When she left the office after each visit, she said, in her most sincere voice and with her best intentions, "Dr. Lebowitz, this time I am going to do what you say." Nevertheless, whenever she came back the next time, it was more of the same. When she came in for her last visit before the office closed, she apologized for her lack of medical adherence and hoped that her actions did not contribute to my decision to leave practice. How could anyone get mad at G.D.?

Brainstorming

Some of the patients tried to be resourceful and come up with solutions to help our business problems. One wished that he were Donald Trump and could pay to keep the practice open. I told him that if there were any extra money available, I would give it to my staff in the form of raises, because many of them were quitting, due to the financial constraints of the DEC. I desperately needed their assistance in treating the countless patients with diabetes and other endocrine disorders. I could not have been successful in practice without my staff, as I emphasized to them many times over the years.

Others were equally creative. Some offered to come live with me or for me to come live with them. A neighbor of mine with diabetes, who was also my patient, offered to come to my house for his quarterly checkups. Others had more elaborate ideas for sustaining the practice, like making it similar to a BJ's wholesale store, where you would have to pay a membership fee each year to come to the practice. This patient actually did all the calculations for me with regard to how much money the BJ's idea could generate. Still others suggested a boutique practice, which could be limited to a few hundred patients. There would be no insurance involved. Rather, each person would pay a flat yearly fee that would cover all their care and the office costs. It was tempting, but I know myself: I could not in good conscience limit my practice to only those who could afford it. How could I sleep at night knowing that I could have helped someone, but would not, because of inability to pay?

Bonds Broken

The patients who really made me do my best waffling about my decision, "to leave, or not to leave," were those sad ones who wept in my office. P.K. was a fortyish-year-old woman, whom I had gotten to know very well over the years. She had a large thyroid goiter with multiple aspirated nodules. Her tests came back equivocal. We could not rule out cancer. After several long discussions, we decided to have the gland removed surgically, which was done several years ago with no adverse event, no negative consequences, and, thankfully, no cancer.

Since we had developed a tight relationship, and since I had become familiar with her son and his rare illness, she liked to come to the office once a year to have her thyroid hormone levels checked and, maybe, just to chat. One day, at a routine visit, after our usual discussion I began to examine her. Although she felt well, her pulse was only thirty! An electrocardiogram (EKG) showed that she was in complete heart block, a potentially fatal condition that could kill her at any moment. Long story short, she had a pacemaker implanted that very day. Each time she came to the office after that, she thanked me for saving her life. On our last visit, she cried, recalling all that we had been through with her thyroid and the heart block.

Simarlily, J.W. cried at her last office visit. We had first met when I was a first-year endocrine fellow in 1989. She was a thirty-year-old mother of five, working full-time, hospitalized for profound exhaustion and unexplained episodes of passing out. Many physicians, including an internist, cardiologist, neurologist, and psychiatrist had evaluated her and thought she was suffering from panic attacks. Nevertheless, she was not convinced. Reluctantly her attending physician called for an endocrine consultation. (One of my mentors had an expression, "The diagnostically destitute always come to the endocrinologist," which means, "If something is wrong, and there is no other diagnosis, then it must be hormonal.")

After meeting J.W., something was telling me that she was right, that her symptoms were not emotional, and that there was an underlying physical, medical condition causing them. Indeed, she had an unusual condition called "mast cell activation syndrome without mast cell proliferation." She responded exquisitely well to the rather simple treatment and never had any of these symptoms again. She also wept at our last office visit as she recounted our first meetings.

E.J. might have been the hardest person to leave. I had known him since my earliest days in practice. At that time he had more medical problems than God had ever intended for one person to have: diabetes with retinopathy, neuropathy, nephropathy, high blood pressure, high cholesterol, hypothyroidism, coronary and peripheral artery disease, chronic atrial fibrillation, advanced arthritis, degenerative disc disease, and bilateral carpal tunnel syndrome. It was actually quicker to list his good organs instead of the diseased ones.

In spite of these maladies, E.J. was typically upbeat and positive when he came for his office visits, which always lasted longer than the scheduled time, because there was much to review and fix. We developed an instant rapport. I looked forward to seeing him and discussing not only his medical conditions but also his views on life and the world. He shared with me his little secrets, like having a keg of beer stowed away in his garage for a little afternoon or evening delight.

Over the years, E.J.'s medical conditions deteriorated, despite my trying to optimize his medications and treatments. His kidneys were failing; he required coronary bypass surgery and surgery for lower extremity claudication. Arthritis intensified in his knees and back. He had multiple operative procedures, even going to Florida for an experimental back procedure, because the conventional procedure done locally did not improve his intractable pains. I helped to make all these cumbersome arrangements for him. His diabetic neuropathy progressed, despite maximizing his glycemia. It became difficult for him, not only to walk to his garage for beer, but also even to hold his glass to drink it. It was obvious that E.J.'s condition was worse at each office visit, which made our last one together the most difficult.

I do not have a crystal ball. If I did, then I might be

tempted to use it all the time. At our last visit together, it was clear that E.J.'s life expectancy could not be too much longer. His voice was soft, he was relegated to a wheelchair, his hands had lost all their musculature — a sign of advanced neuropathy — and he looked ashen and weak. As we said our good-byes, E.J. broke down and cried. I held back my own tears until I left the exam room and was in the privacy of my own office. Although I had thought all along that the "other team" of the insurance companies and the policy makers were the villains, maybe I was really the villain. How could I leave all these patients, people who had trusted and relied on me through the years?

Patient Feedback

When, out of curiosity, I asked patients, during our last visits together, what was it that made them want to continue with my care, they all said the same things: I spent time with them. I genuinely listened to them. They trusted my judgments. I restored their faith in doctors. They always knew that I had their best interests at heart. For example, T.A., a very heavy African American with type 2 diabetes, on insulin and with paranoid schizophrenia, said to me when I was trying to invigorate him to take better care of himself, "Doc, sometimes I think you care more about me than I care about me."

Some patients, with whom I did not feel I was connecting and who just continued to see me, because it was convenient, or because there was too much inertia to change, said the same. Frankly, I had underestimated the impact I had on people's lives. That made my leaving even more difficult for me. "Maybe I am making the wrong decision?" I continually questioned myself: "Maybe I should stay. How can I possibly leave my patients now when there is not only a shortage of endocrinologists but I am at the peak of my game? The situation is really not that bad."

The Acceptance Phase

Finally, my wife asked me, regarding my continued consternation with leaving, "What is the problem?" I responded, "Who will take care of the patients?"

"For now, there are still very good doctors in Central New York," she said, "Your patients will be well taken care of." She was right. With that, I became even more steadfast with my decision to leave. In many respects, I felt like I had gone through all five stages of dying as described in Elisabeth Kübler-Ross's 1969 book, *On Death and Dying*: denial, anger, depression, bargaining, and finally acceptance. The main difference was that I was accepting that I was going to live, not die.

As I rehashed my reasons for leaving with each and every patient that came to the office during the last five months of practice, about twenty times each day, I began to gain energy from most of their empathetic responses: "I do not blame you for leaving." "Why put up with all the crap?" "The insurance companies have too much power and they are greedy. Look at the CEOs' salaries and benefits." "Our premiums are rising and we get less service and more aggravation despite our increased costs." "The politicians are not helping at all and they are on the take as well from the insurance and pharmaceutical lobbyists."

The cost of health care may put my whole business out of business — we cannot compete with companies overseas who do not have the same health care costs. It is all so unfair to American doctors and American patients. Why would any of our best and brightest students go into medicine anymore? There are so many other ways to make a living. The future of our country's health care looks bleak. It was infinitely clear to me that I was not the only one experiencing pain and suffering caused by the American health care system.

Chapter Eight

What I Miss Most About
the Practice of Medicine

Being A Sleuth

I was usually the one asking the questions, but this time, one of my patients asked me, "Doc, what do you think you'll miss most from not practicing medicine?" I paused for a moment, stroked my chin, considered the many possibilities, and then answered him as best I could.

I realized that I would miss being in the exam room, where I was on the prowl, a vigilant medical detective always looking for clues for any asymptomatic conditions or unusual diagnoses that may be present, always trying to solve someone's riddle. I gave him examples. An elderly long-time patient, whom I saw every three months, had mental retardation and stable diabetes. During one office visit he got up from his chair in the exam room to go onto the examining table. He had a new shuffling gait. Examination revealed cogwheel rigidity and, as the famous football announcer John Madden would say — BOOM! — I diagnosed him with Parkinson's disease.

Another patient, a prominent judge, was in for a routine follow-up on his osteoporosis. He was complaining of night sweats over the previous few weeks and had just seen his internist and cardiologist. He was typically a minimizer, so, whenever he complained about anything, I took it very seriously. He had a harsh heart murmur, which sounded a bit different from what it had in the past. I did blood cultures and — BOOM! — I found that he had endocarditis, a life-threatening bacterial infection of one of his heart valves.

Still another was a healthy middle-aged man referred to me by my neighbor for a general checkup. "I have no complaints," he said, "I just want to establish with a new doctor." After a relatively casual conversation, I began examining him.

As a habit, and trying to be systematic, I always checked for a spleen tip when I did the abdominal exam, never expecting it to be abnormal, especially in an otherwise healthy individual. But this one in a million times — BOOM! — He had a large spleen, which turned out to be a consequence of cirrhosis of the liver. He was a "social drinker." His story did not have a happy conclusion. After surgery for a liver transplant, he died.

I will miss the person who came in with a complicated history, had seen other providers, and had gone without a formal diagnosis other than, "It's in your head." Mrs. P. complained of relentless fatigue, loss of appetite, and weight loss. She had significant back pains, for which she received multiple steroid shots in her spine. Other physicians had postulated that her symptoms were due to either her pain medications or depression, which is commonly associated with chronic pain. They were wrong. As it turned out, she had developed adrenal insufficiency, a consequence of the multiple steroid injections. Mrs. P. responded beautifully after I treated her with the appropriate adrenal replacement hormones.

Like shooting a basketball and hearing the swish when the ball went through the net, for me it never got old when patients with obesity and subsequent diabetes, hypertension, and hyperlipidemia felt considerably better and were able to discontinue all their medications after they lost weight by dieting and exercising. In my experience as an endocrinologist, there are three things in life that are 100 per cent guaranteed to happen: First, nobody gets out of here alive — even Methuselah died and he was 969 years old. Second, until we die, and maybe even afterward, we have to pay taxes. Third, anyone who diets, exercises, and loses weight will feel better.

I never got tired of cases in which patients came to see me with profound symptoms due to definable problems, like new onset type 1 diabetes with the profuse drinking, urinating, weight loss, blurred vision, and fatigue that was treatable with the wonderful new insulins that have become available. I received so much satisfaction from their dramatic responses to treatment, as all their symptoms resolved in a relatively short period. I also felt great joy when patients with symptomatic

overactive thyroid glands (thyrotoxicosis), suffering from un-
intentional weight loss, tremors, palpitations, and insomnia,
had their symptoms clear up after being given the appropriate
therapy. Some of these patients enjoyed the weight loss and
asked if it might be possible just to treat all the other thyro-
toxic symptoms except the weight loss. Sorry!

Being appreciated by the patients whom I helped
through particularly difficult times was something I knew I
would miss. I assisted many pregnant women with diabetes
by maintaining phone contact with them several times a week
during their pregnancies, in addition to their usual office visits.
We were all so grateful and relieved when they delivered
healthy babies. One man with a prolactin producing pituitary
tumor complicated by pituitary apoplexy, a sudden hemorrhage
into the tumor, was subsequently, with the help of medications I prescribed, able to impregnate his wife. In gratitude
they named their little boy "Mitchell," my real name.

The Art of Medicine

What I liked most about being a physician was using all my
skills, some learned in medical school, others learned after
years of experience as a clinician. Other skills that I found
helpful were either innate or based on my own life's experiences. Sometimes I needed all these learned and experiential
abilities and more to manage a certain situation. The following
cases were not found in textbooks. Equally important, my experience had not provided me adequate preparation for them.
Yet, as these patients' physician, I needed to figure out the
best way to manage them..

A forty-eight-year-old male patient had hypogonado-
trophic hypogonadism, a low testosterone level, due to pituitary gland insufficiency. His hypothalamus and/or pituitary
gland had stopped making not only the hormones that stimu-
lated his testicles to make testosterone, the male hormone,
but also the hormones that allowed for sperm production. In
short, he was infertile. Therefore, when he told me that his

wife was pregnant I was caught off guard. I am sure I looked dumbfounded, because I frequently wear my emotions on my face. I thought of many different things to say, such as, "You may want to consider having the baby's DNA checked," but all I could say was, "Congratulations!"

Analogous to that situation was the one in which a middle-aged man requested Viagra so that he could have an adulterous affair. I begrudgingly gave him the prescription, with the understanding that he not call me in the middle of the night to tell me that it had worked.

I had a limited practice with transgender patients. They were some of the nicest, most grateful, and compliant patients I have ever had. Years ago a therapist referred a sixteen-year-old girl to my office. She was interested in becoming a sixteen-year-old boy. I had concerns that sixteen was too young to make such an irreversible decision. This patient had a complicated family life. Although her mother was supportive and accompanied her to the office visits, she was estranged from her father. There were many reasons, including legal, ethical, and moral, that made me feel that this was not the correct course for her at the time and I declined her request for treatment. To be certain about my decision, I obtained an opinion from the ethics committee at the local hospital where I also practiced. I was thankful when the members of the committee agreed with my decision. In 2007 I learned that this girl, then in her twenties, was still a "she."

Genetic Testing Meets Clinical Medicine

Genetic testing presented new kinds of challenges. A woman asked my advice on testing her younger son for the likelihood that he could develop type 1 diabetes. Her older son already was stricken with the disease. In many respects she just wanted to be reassured that her younger son was not going to get the condition. She knew that there were no treatments available to prevent him from getting diabetes even if the tests came back positive, although there are ongoing studies in this direction. She decided to have him tested anyway. Much to her despair, his tests were very positive. Her tears could not prevent him from developing diabetes just a few weeks later.

Another gene testing situation had a happier ending. I took care of a very large family that had an uncommon disease called medullary thyroid cancer (MTC). It had claimed the lives of several of their family members. Thanks to modern genetics, and after an enormous amount of work by a physician/geneticist in Michigan, the family's atypical gene underlying the condition was finally identified. I had the whole family tested and two of the teenage sons' tests came back positive. Should I have recommended prophylactic removal of their thyroid glands, which would have eliminated their chances of developing this potentially life-threatening condition, but incurring the risks of this surgical procedure in asymptomatic teenagers? Or, should I have waited and followed them "expectedly" (the medical euphemism for "Do nothing and see what happens")? What would you have suggested?

I used "Lebowitz's Rule # 1": Always err on the side of safety. I thought it would be safer to take the thyroid glands out now than to have the boys show up at my door one day when they were adults with metastatic MTC, an incurable disease. The procedures went fine, without complications. Now all they need to do is take their regular doses of thyroid hormone replacement and have their thyroid hormone levels checked about once a year — a better tradeoff indeed.

Trying to Hold Back My Tears — The End of Life

Some of the challenges that my patients and I faced related to end-of-life issues. One of my eighty-two-year-old patients, a survivor of the Holocaust, replied when I asked him how he was doing, "Doc, the parts are made to wear out." We all know that no one gets out of here alive, but how different people deal with death is of great interest to me.

Ms. W. was in her fifties with diabetes and all its complications, including kidney failure that required dialysis. During the years that I treated her she suffered heart attacks, strokes, and fatal pancreatic cancer. She was in the hospital for the last days of her life. In spite of all the medical hardships that she had encountered over the years, and with very few social relationships left to her, she did not want to die. She cried to me every day when I saw her on rounds, but her fate was cast and her day came. Then it was my turn to cry.

Other patients — miraculously — accept their fate. Mr. O. also had renal failure. He was receiving hemodialysis three times per week. Hemodialysis requires two very large bore needles to be placed into an enlarged blood vessel called a fistula, which is constructed in the arm by a surgeon. Each dialysis treatment lasts around four hours, not including transportation back and forth to the center or the time necessary to recuperate from each treatment. People often feel lousy, tired, worn out, after their dialysis treatments. Travel to another dialysis center away from one's own is occasionally necessary, but is problematic and hassle-laden, because arrangements need to be made well in advance — as if anyone on dialysis actually feels well enough to travel. After being on dialysis for years, Mr. O. had had enough. He talked with me about stopping dialysis and letting nature take its course. I never saw him so content as in the days after he decided to stop treatments and before he passed away.

Mrs. F. had also had enough. She was in her late seventies and had very advanced medical problems. Her parents had gone to sleep one night and did not wake up, but she complained to me that for her, "Death is taking so long."

Mr. S., in his late fifties, was a singer, songwriter, and fun-loving international traveler with a contagious smile and laugh. He was a very likeable guy who, sad to say, had smoked too many cigarettes and developed lung cancer. When it was discovered, it was already widely metastatic. His only treatment option was chemotherapy to palliate, not to cure the disease. I wanted him to go for the treatment. Maybe I was being selfish, because I loved seeing him in my office and hearing his optimistic views of life and his stories of world travels, but he had other plans. "Mickey," he told me, "I've had a good

life. I'm not taking any treatments and I'm ready to go." There
was a huge void in my practice, and my life, after he died.

It Was Not All Seriousness — The Lighter Side of Medicine

But the practice of medicine was not always business and
drama. I love to laugh and there were countless comedic moments in the exam room. The comments by the guys prior to,
during, and after their prostate exams could fill an entire book
by themselves: "But we haven't even had our first date yet."
"You're going to use a glove, aren't you? And lubrication?"
"I'd like a second opinion; can you use two fingers?" "I'll be
suspicious if you put your hands on each of my shoulders."
"Do you see the sign down there that says 'Exit Only'?"
"How was it for you?" "You want a smoke now that's its
over?" In the "end," I would just tell the guys to assume the
position, bend over, and get enlightened to the fact that it
would hurt them more than it would hurt me.

Others came up with interesting, original ideas, such
as the woman who thought that we should have all come
with instructions on how we work and how to fix us if we
break. "Not that the male doctors would read the instructions
anyway," she said.

"What would be so bad if we were born old and died
young?" one of my senior patients commented. "That way we
could have the physical abilities and maybe even some money
to do all the things that we learned over the years and, if you
think about it, why would it matter? Either way we have to
have our butts wiped and we have to be fed. So what's the
difference?"

One guy, who had gone through multiple surgeries,
thought that we should have been born with zippers so we
would not have to be cut open for each operation.

A young woman's arms would fall asleep when she lay
on them in bed each night. She just did not know what to do
with them or where to put them while she slept. But she had
an idea. She thought it would be perfect if she could just un-

screw her arms, take them off while she slept, then reconnect them in the morning.

It always amused me when a patient came in complaining of a cough, saying, "You want to hear it? Listen." Then he or she would proceed to ... cough.

Sex stories also abounded, but not your typical ones. One of my octogenarians had sex with his equally aged, widowed sister-in-law. He wished that he had been with her when she was younger, because "she was quite good." One of my seventy-year-old patients boasted that he had had sex every Sunday with the same woman for years. He went to her house for lunch, they spoke very little, then they did it. He explained how both looked forward to the routine. Another male, a bit younger, had retrograde ejaculation as a consequence of a urological procedure. This meant that when he ejaculated the semen would go into his bladder rather than come out through his penis. He did not mind it, because "it's less messy when I masturbate."

There were many comedic moments. One patient brought in a large toenail that had fallen off years ago. He was not sure if it was important but he thought that someday it might help a future doctor care for him. So he saved it in an airtight bag, preserved for time eternal. But, other than being funny, it served no medical purpose.

When I was a third-year student on the urology rotation I walked into an exam room where the patient, an elderly male, was waiting to be seen. I began to introduce myself, somewhat shyly, as I was still very green around patients. I said to him, "Hello, Mr. So-and-So, my name is Mickey Lebowitz. I am a third-year medical student and ..." Before I could say another word, he jumped out of his chair, pulled down his slacks and underpants so that his boys were now hanging out. He certainly caught me off guard. I was not used to any guy, especially one whom I had barely met, just whipping out his personals, but I composed myself enough and urged him to "put those things away" until we at least had a chance to talk.

Also as a third-year medical student, I was on call at the Acute Psychiatric Center. A new patient came in and the resident suggested that I see her first. When I went into the room the woman looked like she had escaped from *Night of the Living Dead*. Her hair was gray and scraggly. Her skin was as pale as it could be in a person who was still alive. Her teeth were cracked, angulated, and vampirish. Her fingernails were grotesquely long with black stuff underneath them. She was scantily dressed in black rags that barely passed for clothes. She looked at me with a terror in her eyes like I had never seen. Then she screeched at the top of her lungs, "I want to die!" I did what any kind, caring, empathetic, compassionate student doctor would do ... I freakin' ran out of the room! I never did well with scary movies and this was even scarier. I ran to the resident, who cracked up seeing me hyperventilate, sweat from my brow, and have all the color drained from my face. He asked, "What? Did you just see a ghost?" Maybe I did. I was definitely out of my league. I let the varsity doctor handle the rest of that case.

Talking about the varsity, my friend, the team doctor for Syracuse University athletic teams, invited me to attend an SU football game with him one Saturday afternoon, including going into the locker room and standing on the sidelines. As I was standing there, innocently enjoying the game, it dawned on me that I was a hormone doctor standing with the football team in plain sight of everyone in the Carrier Dome. Could I then, in this era of performance-enhancing drugs, possibly be misconstrued by some as performing an act of impropriety?

I convinced myself otherwise and went on enjoying the game expecting that no one would really notice. WRONG! As I walked through the hospital doors the following Monday, I was greeted by many who wanted to know why the hormone doctor was on the sidelines with the football team. Was I the new Brian McNamee or was I clean?

My Patients Were People, Not Just Diseases

What I will also miss is getting to know some wonderful people besides just their medical conditions. I always loved when they brought in their artwork, photographs, or writings. I looked forward to hearing stories about their vacation trips or nice events in their lives, like birthdays, anniversaries, or having new grandchildren. Some of my storytellers, especially the seniors, lived alone, isolated, and saw me not only for medical reasons but also as a friend and confidante.

It was therapeutic for them, as good as any pill, having pleasant face-to-face conversations with someone they liked, and telling their story, rather than just listening to a voice on the TV or radio. It was therapeutic for me as well. Their stories constantly reminded me that I was not taking care of diabetes and hypertension. I was taking care of people who had diabetes and hypertension. I knew that I had connected with them when, at the end of our time together, they gave me big hugs, kisses, or genuine handshakes. I truly enjoyed hearing their stories and learning more about their previous lives, such as Mr. D., a salt-of-the-earth type of guy, eighty-eight years old, a World War II combat veteran, very active in war veterans groups. He routinely went to elementary and middle schools to teach our younger generations about his experiences, lest they forget the sacrifices that many have made for them to continue to have their freedoms. People like him made me stand at attention and feel proud that I was able to serve him back.

Maybe There Is Something More I Can Do to Serve My Patients

Although there was much that I would miss from practicing medicine, there was also much that I would not. I had made lists to review the pros and the cons of staying versus leaving. I talked about it with my wife, my parents, my friends, and frankly anyone else who would listen. I thought about it day, night, and frequently through the night. Should I leave? Yes. Could I leave? Yes. Would I leave? Yes. I was done complaining and whining and about the inequities. We needed changes before more of us left. Maybe I could contribute somehow toward bringing about these changes, now that I was unburdened from the endless demands of being in full-time practice.

So, although it was very difficult at times, I stayed the course.

I looked forward to my last day in practice. It seemed like it would never come. I felt like each day lasted a week and each week lasted a year. I limped to the finish line. Whatever staff we had left were quitting — understandably. They were looking for new jobs before we closed on October 31, 2007. The staff that remained — there was no one to bring up from the minor leagues as the franchise was being shut down — tried hard to fill in, even though overloaded with work and responsibility.

I raised my level of diligence and thoroughness even higher during those last few months in practice. I was concerned that something might get missed with the patients, which could result in a disasater for them. I did not think that a patient, a judge, or a jury would be very sympathetic if I were to use the fact that we had inadequate numbers of nurses or the fact that we were going out of business as an excuse for having missed a diagnosis that resulted in harm to a patient. Also, and most importantly, the last thing I wanted was to have a patient suffer any negative consequences from my practice closing. I certainly did not want to wake up in the middle of the night sometime in December 2007 saying, "Oh geez, I forgot to change Mrs. So-and-So's medication. I hope she's OK."

Still, many days I felt like a villain for quitting and leaving "my team": my patients and my colleagues. Many other days I felt like a victim of an unfair game, in which the sides were not even, and which was nothing like I grew up playing in the streets of Brooklyn. Now the "other team" made all the rules, bullied us, and expected us to play their way, all while they took advantage of our altruism, commitment, dedication, and obligation to our patients. I would do a lot of things for "my team," but I would not do that.

My Last Day of Medical Practice

You may ask, "What really happened the last day of practice?" Did my fantasy come true? Were there bands playing? Speeches from satisfied patients? News cameras and beat writers looking for exit interviews? The answers were: No, No, No, and No. I saw my last patient on a Friday afternoon, at 2:50 p.m., October 26, 2007. She was someone I had treated for almost as long as I was in practice. She brought gifts, blew bubbles in the exam room — really! — and gave me a nice card.

After we said our good-byes, I dictated my last notes, finished reviewing my last charts, received hugs and kind words from my residual staff, and walked out the side door. No band, no cameras, no speeches, and not one patient waiting to grab hold of my leg to try to get me to stay as I walked to my car. It was a surreal moment and, like many moments during the previous several months, I felt like I was having an out of body experience, as if I was watching a movie ... of me.

That night I took my usual nightly walk with my wife. We went out to dinner at our favorite Thai restaurant, where the atmosphere was analogous to eating in someone's unfinished basement. In short, nothing special, just another day, although I admit we treated ourselves to a McDonald's McFlurry for dessert ... with the M&Ms. Maybe, after all these years, it just had not yet set in that I was not going to see patients again the following Monday.

Chapter Nine

The American Health Care System is Sick

The rest of this book details many of the issues that I faced, and that physicians in private or small group practice still face daily trying to survive the American health care system. I hope that defining these issues may help to find the best direction for change, if change does ever occur.

A Band-Aid Will Not Work — It Just Covers the Wound

The intensive care doctor stands at the bedside of a critically ill patient lying motionless in her ICU bed. She is intubated, attached to a ventilator where a whooshing sound is made with every inhalation and exhalation. The heart monitor beeps with each beat of her heart, although the beeps are starting to slow down, a sign of impending death. He questions himself, "What is wrong with this patient? Why is she dying?"

He quickly reviews her chart for the history then examines her. He next checks the ventilator settings before returning to the chart to review all her laboratory data, EKGs, and x-ray reports. His assessment: She is volume overloaded. There is too much fluid in her body. She is literally drowning. But why is that? From the studies, he thinks to himself, she had a heart attack. That left her heart weak and unable to pump her blood out to her other organs. The fluid backs up into her lungs, causing pulmonary edema. With fluid in her lungs, oxygen cannot adequately get into her body and she cannot breathe out the carbon dioxide and other wastes. She requires being on a ventilator. Fluid that normally returns to her heart also backs up into her legs, causing massive edema, and into her abdomen. She looks like she has a beer belly, even as she lies flat in bed.

With a weakened heart her other organs are starved for oxygen. Her kidneys and liver begin to show ill effects with abnormal enzymes and limited urine output. Her hands and feet are turning blue, mottled, and cold to the touch. She is pale, associated with the anemia, and there is blood in her stool. The doctor again thinks to himself, "What do I need to do to help this woman?" He quickly puts together all the pieces of the puzzle.

He thinks to himself, "I cannot fix the excess fluid in her body without fixing her liver and kidneys; I cannot fix her lungs, liver, or kidneys until I fix her heart; I cannot fix her heart until I fix the anemia; and I cannot fix the anemia until I find the cause of her gastrointestinal bleeding." He knows he does not have much time, because the patient is dying.

To help this woman, the doctor needs to understand the entire case. He cannot fix just one organ and hope that all the other organs will improve and that the patient will survive. He completely understands that all the systems are connected to each other, like a giant web. The same is true with the American health care system in the early twenty-first century.

Our health care system is also in the ICU. It is terminally sick. It needs a thorough assessment and treatment. Putting a Band-Aid, Steri-Strip, splint, or cast on one of the problems will not fix the entire system.

Taiwan's health care system was in similar disorder in the 1980s. People who could pay received health care while those who could not pay did not. They cured their health care system's sickness by studying other health care systems in the world and taking the best pieces of each to treat their own. With the changes that *they* were willing to make, *they* resuscitated *their* system, so that every Taiwanese citizen could receive health care. If the Taiwanese had the will, desire, and fortitude to fix their problem, why should America not do it too?

One of my patients — let's call him Jim — asked me before I left practice to identify for him the problems that needed to be addressed to fix our failing medical system. Like a boil that had been festering and now was ready to burst I said to him, "I thought no one would ever ask. Do you have a few ... HOURS?"

The Big Picture

According to IOM data from 2004 and World Health Organization (WHO) assessments, America is the only industrialized nation in the world that does not have health care coverage for all its citizens, despite spending more per capita on health care than any other nation. The WHO's *World Health Statistics 2008* reported that in 2006 the United Kingdom spent $3361, Germany $3669, Canada $3912, France $4056, Denmark $4828, Switzerland $5878, Norway $6267, Monaco $6343, and Luxembourg $6610, while the U.S. spent $6714, all per capita. Sixteen per cent of all the money our country spends, our gross domestic product (GDP), is spent on health care. That percentage may be over nineteen by 2017, if federal predictions from the Centers for Medicare and Medicaid Services (CMS) are accurate. In actual amount, the CMS have determined that 2.1 trillion dollars was spent in 2006 either trying to prevent our citizens from getting sick or, more commonly and more costly, treating them when they did. The National Coalition on Health Care (NCHC) has predicted that this amount will double by 2016. The amount of money spent on health care significantly outpaced both inflation and wages between 2001 and 2006. Pamela L. Moore's "The 2006 Fee Schedule Survey: Power to the Payers" in the January 2007 online issue of *Physicians Practice* <www.physicianspractice.com/index/fuseaction/articles.details/articleID/933.htm> showed that health care premiums increased 65.8 per cent, worker's earnings 18.2 per cent, and inflation 16.4 per cent. But the money is not spent equally, as some people receive excellent health care while others get none.

Forty-seven million people in our country do not have health insurance and, likely as a consequence of these uninsured people not seeking or obtaining medical care, the WHO in 2000 ranked us thirty-seventh in the world for performance and seventy-second in overall level of health out of 191 member nations. We rank forty-sixth in the world for infant mortality and fiftieth for life expectancy, according to *CIA World Factbook* estimates for 2009. These figures are getting worse.

Families USA, a national consumer group that analyzes data from the IOM, the Urban Institute, and other authoritative sources, announced on its Web site <www.familiesusa.org/issues/uninsured/publications/dying-for-coverage.html> that lack of health insurance caused about 18,000 deaths in 2000 and 22,000 in 2006. These are more deaths than occur each year from homicide. In general, the uninsured tend to be sicker and die younger because they either go without preventive care or delay care if they do become ill.

Even people with insurance suffer. More than half of all the bankruptcies each year in the U.S. are the result of medical bills; and three quarters of those filers had medical insurance but could not afford the deductibles, co-pays, or medications. David Cay Johnston wrote in his book, *Free Lunch: How the Wealthiest Americans Enrich Themselves at Government Expense (and Stick You With the Bill)* (New York: Penguin, 2007), p. 212, "No one in the modern world ever goes bankrupt because of medical bills, except in the United States of America."

In 2005, about a quarter of Americans with insurance did not fill prescriptions, go for recommended treatments, or see a medical provider when they were sick, according to the Commonwealth Fund's 2005 "Biennial Health Insurance Survey," online at <www.commonwealthfund.org/Content/Surveys/2005/2005-Biennial-Health-Insurance-Survey.aspx>. As a curiosity, I did my own research by looking in our local paper, each week for several weeks, for the number of people who had financial judgments against them of more than $1000, and almost half of the hundreds of those people were in default to a medical institution, such as a hospital.

Business owners are also feeling the pain. They are having a difficult time financially competing with other companies, especially those based overseas, who do not have the added expense of paying full or partial health insurance premiums for their employees, because they operate in countries where there are national health plans. The number of American businesses that offer health insurance to their employees is decreasing steadily, going from 63.6 per cent in 2000 to 59.5 per cent in 2005, according to data from Physicians for a

National Health Program (PNHP). Some foreign companies, Toyota for example, chose to set up some operations in Canada instead of in the U.S., at least in part due to the cost of American health care. On the flipside, American employees often stay in unsatisfying jobs as hostages to the health insurance they receive from their employers.

Despite these negative facts and statistics, some still defend our American health care system as the best in the world and point out, anecdotally, how kings, princes, sheiks, and even dictators come to the U.S. for health care. Well sure, America has the best doctors and medical and surgical facilities in the world, and those rich foreign potentates can afford American health care; but that does not mean that ordinary Americans can afford American health care. Some American citizens actually leave our country to seek medical care outside our borders. But such flight is because of easier access to care abroad, not because foreign countries offer better quality of care.

The term "medical tourism" has been popularized by travel agents who have facilitated arrangements for Americans, many without or with only limited insurance, to travel overseas for more affordable treatments, such as elective surgical or dental procedures. Countries such as China, Thailand, Colombia, India, and Israel are among the destinations of our citizens seeking less expensive, yet efficacious treatments. Imagine that to get on a plane, travel halfway around the world, stay in a hotel, and get an operation is less expensive than to purchase health insurance here in our own country.

Jim, who had asked me to define the issues with the American health care system and had been listening intently as I described to him "The Big Picture," was just about to fall asleep as I droned on about increasing costs, the number of uninsureds, and our low health care rankings compared with the rest of the world. But just before his eyelids completely covered his eyes, he sprang back to wakefulness to ask another poignant question: "So, Doc, how does this affect you as a physician?" I responded, "Let me explain it to you by describing one case as an example."

An Example of the Impact of the Health Care System on the Individual Physician

Mrs. H. came to my office a day after she was discharged from the hospital, where she had been admitted one week prior with a fractured pelvis from a fall. She was a frail, elderly woman with totally gray hair, weighed about 100 pounds, and wore dark oversized glasses to shield her impaired eyes from the light. Mrs. H. had had diabetes for over forty years and, despite five injections of insulin per day, her blood sugars were all over the place. Given her impaired vision, her husband would draw up the insulin into a syringe, but she injected it herself. As a consequence of her diabetes, she had neuropathy, which expressed itself most profoundly when she stood up and her blood pressure dropped. To make the situation even more challenging, she had high blood pressure when she sat or lay down in bed, which made adjusting her blood pressure medications almost impossible. She also had active coronary artery disease, a history of stroke, high cholesterol, osteoporosis, and progressive dementia.

Her husband accompanied her that day in my office. Although she was told to follow up with me as soon as possible after she was discharged, I had no hospital records, and I was never informed by the hospitalist who had treated her in the hospital that she had ever even been admitted. Therefore, I relied on her husband to update me about the events that led to her admission.

He told me that, just before he called the ambulance to take Mrs. H. to the hospital, he saw her crawling around on the floor as if she were looking for something. She seemed more confused than usual, but he was not sure how she actually had come to be on the floor, whether she had done so intentionally, had fallen, or had briefly lost consciousness. She was in significant pain when he tried to lift her, so he called the ambulance and they brought her to the hospital. She was later diagnosed with a fractured pelvis.

So here I was, one week later, without any hospital records and no information from the providers who had treated her in the hospital, trying to figure out what had happened. Did she lose consciousness because she had had a stroke? Did she have a cardiac event such as a heart attack or arrhythmia? Was a low blood sugar reaction the cause of her increased confusion? Did she suffer a low blood pressure episode, due to her diabetic neuropathy, when she tried to stand up? Or did she maybe just trip and fall because of her poor vision? How did she break her pelvis? She was on osteoporosis medications. Was she actually taking this medicine? I needed the answers to these questions to try to prevent whatever caused her problem from happening again.

I had many decisions to make. Should I add medications to prevent her from having another possible heart attack or stroke? Should I adjust her insulin to prevent her from having another possible low blood sugar reaction? Should I reduce her blood pressure medication to prevent her from having low blood pressure when she stood up, even if it meant having higher blood pressure when she sat down or lay flat? Did she break her pelvis because of the fall, or because she was not taking the osteoporosis medication adherently, or because she had another problem affecting her bone density, such as vitamin D deficiency or thyrotoxicosis? I had only a short time to make these decisions — and make them accurately. How would I do it?

I would use the factors that were in my control to help Mrs. H., such as my knowledge base from all my reading, studying, and teaching on the different subjects, as well as my experiences and past judgments; and I would do so in an empathetic, compassionate way. After I spoke with the patient and her husband, I examined her. I assessed her symptoms and measured her blood pressure lying, sitting, and standing, to see whether it decreased with change in position and, if so, by how much. I also did a complete mental status and neurological examination.

Next, I needed to take into account the factors over which I had no control, such as what her insurance might pay if I needed to do any tests or prescribe any new medications, how much time my staff would need to sit on the phone to get the test approved, and how many forms they or I would need to fill out to obtain a new medication.

Since Mr. and Mrs. H. are on fixed incomes as retirees, I had to take into account their co-pays and deductibles for the tests or medications that I suggested. I also needed to try to determine what the patient's and her husband's expectations were for the treatment and prognosis, all the while keeping in mind that I did not want to make any mistakes in trying to fix these complex problems, mistakes that might lead to harming the patient or even to a lawsuit.

Also, I needed to do the best I could without any communication — whether directly by conversation or indirectly by written reports — from the physicians who had treated her in the hospital. Communication among physicians is often less than optimal and may significantly add to the challenge of giving a patient the best possible care without duplicating tests. In "Who's Calling the Shots?" in the April 2008 *More* magazine, Shannon Brownlee reported an estimate that eleven per cent of lab tests and x-rays are duplicated each year, at significant expense to the system, because neither the physician nor the patient knew that the studies had been done already, or because they did not yet have the results available, or because no one bothered to find out.

My practice did not have a fully functional electronic medical records (EMR) system, but we were trying to move in that direction and we did have e-prescriptions. Catherine DesRoches, Eric Campbell, *et al.*, reported in the July 3, 2008, *NEJM* that only four per cent of medical offices nationwide had complete EMR and only thirteen per cent had even a basic EMR system. The cost in both time and money to start a completely paperless system is prohibitive for most private practices. On the other hand, the VA EMR is the best in the country. All its patient records go back to the 1990s, include all diagnostic and imaging tests and results, and make available all physician and ancillary care notes, regardless of where in the country each patient was seen. Unlike that system, my computer system had no direct interface with the local hospital just a few miles away. Moreover, it would not have had this interface even if it had been maximally functional. I could not access my own patients' hospital records through my system. This is just one unfortunate example of the fragmentation that exists in our nationwide health care "system."

Although the patient wanted to see me instead of her primary care doctor, because she believed that her problems were hormonal and therefore best evaluated by her endocrinologist, I had to make sure, as a consultant, that I would evaluate and resolve only those issues that I thought were in my ballpark, so as not to overstep my boundaries or offend her primary care physician.

I needed to be aware of my own financial interest in this case. I could either order tests that could be done in my office for my profit, benefiting my own self-interest, or I could have my staff spend significant time trying to contact the hospital to get the records, so as possibly to avoid duplication of tests and unnecessary expenses to the patient and the system, which would cost me time and money, because my staff could always be doing other things to help me generate revenue, like being available for me to see more patients.

I also needed to be aware of the pharmaceutical industries' influences on my decisions, whether directly, via sales representatives or pharmaceutical-sponsored publications, or indirectly, from Mr. H., who just had just seen, in one of the diabetes magazines in my waiting room, an advertisement describing the wonderments of the latest and greatest "me-too" medicine.

Physicians are at the Epicenter of the Health Care System

Jim, now completely wide-eyed and awake as I described all these details to him, responded, "Doc, you're at the epicenter of the medical system." Epicenter?! The quarterback, maybe. The point guard, possibly. The catcher, perhaps. But epicenter? I knew the term was associated with earthquakes, but I had never imagined it in connection with being a physician.

So I looked it up in *The American Heritage Dictionary of the English Language* and yes, it gave reference to an earthquake, but definition number two was, "a focal point."

As I thought more about the term that Jim had used to describe the physicians' role in the American health care system, I thought he was quite accurate. Physicians *are* the focal point of the system. We have a unique vantage point to see the issues from all different perspectives. We have enormous responsibilities to the patients, and the patients in turn look back to us for guidance. The payers (the insurance companies, CMS) and the payees (the patients and the business owners) alike look to us to make cost-effective decisions while the pharmaceutical industry tries to entice us to prescribe their expensive medications. The malpractice attorneys keep checks and balances on us. The government tries to regulate the system through us.

Jim looked at me as if I were an enlightened soul, which I certainly am not, and said, "Doc, give me more details of the problems and any solutions." Now the boil burst, as I let go a flow of thoughts, anecdotes, stories, and studies to define the issues as I saw them from my epicentral vantage point, as a physician in the trenches, doing the daily hand-to-hand combat, one case at a time.

But what is most distressing is that, unlike in Taiwan, the issues are essentially the same in 2009 as they were in 1999, 1989, or even 1979, despite stadiums that could be filled with writings about the problems, and despite thousands of exhaustive discussions, meetings, and symposiums. These issues were so upsetting, even back then, that PNHP (15,000 strong in 2008) was founded in 1987 and published its first major proposal in *NEJM* in 1989. Then there was Hillary Clinton's attempt at health care reform in the mid-1990s. From my vantage point, not only are the issues being discussed the same as they were thirty years ago, but, through continued significant and well-heeled resistance to change, the problems have intensified.

Chapter Ten

Time (or, Lack Thereof)

One of my favorite songs is "The Dock of the Bay" by Otis Redding, which is about wasting time. Time is one of the most precious of all commodities. Once it is used, it is gone forever. There is no guarantee that you will ever get any more in the future. Seeing my kids just sitting at the computer *ad infinitum* was *ad nauseum* to me, because I felt that they were wasting what I cherished and wished I had more of: time. When I was in practice, I wished I could, even for one day, just sit on a dock and waste time.

Before Office Hours

While in private practice I felt like every minute of every day was calculated from the time I woke up by my alarm clock at 6:23 a.m., or by my beeper before then if there was a patient in need, until the time I went to sleep, around 10:30 p.m. — after watching my umpteen millionth rerun of *Seinfeld*.

Even the amount of time I slept was calculated. I envied my friend who needed only five hours of sleep each night, compared with my eight. When I broke it down, this meant that he had three hours more each day of awake time, which equalled twenty-one hours more per week, at least eighty-four more per month, and 1095 hours more per year of awake time — 1098 in leap years! That is over forty-five DAYS each year, over a month and a half of Februaries, that he is awake while I am sleeping.

I know this is quirky (although maybe you do the same), but I calculated how much time it took me in the bathroom each morning to shower and shave. My shirts were half-buttoned when they came back from the dry cleaner so I just pulled them over my head while dressing. I calculated my steps and movements around the kitchen while preparing breakfast, so that there were no wasted or backward steps.

Before I gave up my hospital practice in 2004, I used to eat breakfast while walking through the hospital to save time. Whenever possible, I used both my hands simultaneously, hoping to save time, even if it meant just saving seconds. For example, I would use one hand to attach my cell phone and beeper to my belt while using the other to put away my phone charger and put my wallet in my pocket.

My drive to work was also strictly calculated. There was one stop light I had to go through to get to work, eight miles away. I knew that it changed every two minutes, odd minutes that is: 7:19, 7:21, 7:23, etc. It took about ninety seconds to drive from my house to the light. Therefore, depending on what time it was when I left my garage, I could either speed through the side streets to make the light or know that I would miss it and take my time until the next light change.

Once I got on the highway, if I went 74.9 mph (which my state trooper patients told me is the unofficial speed limit I could go without getting a ticket in a 65 mph zone), and if there were no delays for construction, accidents, or weather, I could be at the office at exactly 7:30 a.m., ready to see my first patient. That was when the serious time calculations really went into effect.

Office Hours: Do It With a Smile!

In the exam room, I wanted the patients to feel like I had all the time in the world for them. However, I knew that I had only twenty minutes for each of them. I could not let them see that I was periodically looking at my watch, because people are often offended when they see you checking the time, like you want to get rid of them. I tried not to run past the allotted time, but, in many instances, that was impossible. Most patients had so many physical, emotional, and social problems to discuss that I frequently needed more than the scheduled twenty minutes. Just solving the patients' problems and communicating my opinions back to them was usually achievable, but solving these problems with added time constraints made the tasks much more difficult. I felt like I was playing "Beat the Clock" about twenty times a day. Or maybe it was like "Name That Tune / Make That Diagnosis." I would try to make a diagnosis with as few questions as possible: "You're exhausted? You snore at night? You're overweight? Diagnosis: Sleep apnea. Next problem." — That was no way to deal with people.

If I was running behind schedule and knew that I was keeping the next patient waiting, I felt extra pressure that showed up as tightness in my neck, irritability, and talking even faster than my usual "Brooklyn speed." I dreaded those uncomfortable feelings and tried to suppress them, but they often became obvious, especially to my patients who knew me well, because I typically wore my emotions on my sleeves. The patients would ask if I was OK? Then I felt bad, guilty that I had kept them waiting so long, and spent even more time with them. That would just compound the problem. (I always admired psychiatrists who could end their patient visits, no matter where they were in the conversation, at exactly ten minutes to the hour.) So, I calculated how much time I could spend with each patient doing the history and the physical exam, and still leave time for discussion. Plus, I had to do it all with a smile.

On one particular Monday morning — usually the most stressful time of the week anyway — my first patient, at 7:30 a.m., had fifty minutes worth of problems to tackle in her twenty-minute office visit. She had diabetes being treated with insulin, retinopathy, neuropathy, high blood pressure, high cholesterol, back and leg pains, osteoporosis, hypothyroidism, and depression, to name just a few of her maladies. I knew that the rest of the day would be extra difficult because I was already thirty minutes late for my next appointment. At the end of the visit, which required my maximal concentration and problem-solving skills, I gave her solutions for all her problems. However, she was not satisfied. She said, "Doctor, you aren't smiling today." UUGGHH!!!

Be Quick But Don't Hurry

To be fast yet thorough, I used a system developed by the FPA docs to maximize care and efficiency for my most time-consuming patients, those with diabetes. While I was seeing a patient, I had one of my nurses not only bring the next patient to an open exam room, but also check that patient's blood sugars and blood sugar average, the hemoglobin A1c, with our six-minute tester. Next, the nurse would ask the patient questions and fill out a lengthy form that I had made to update all the pertinent information, such as new problems since the last visit, a review of medications, and a check that I was following all the ADA guidelines, including the patient's last eye, cholesterol, and kidney exams. Because I saw so many people with diabetes, this form was enormously helpful to ensure that each person was receiving appropriate, up-to-date, and recommended treatments. Sometimes the patients blurred together, so that I was uncertain about whether I had asked someone something about care or not. The form helped to make the care consistent. The nurses would then ready the patient for the examination, including asking that shoes and socks be removed so that I could inspect the feet for diabetic neuropathy and otherwise asymptomatic ulcers.

To help with efficiency and accuracy, my nurse stayed in the examining room with me during my time with the patient. While doing the physical examination, I dictated my findings to her, which she transcribed onto the form. She also wrote down the assessment and plan as I told it to the patient. Last, she wrote down the instructions for the patient, as a reminder of what to do after arriving home. (My handwriting is so bad that one of my patients once brought a tape recorder to the office visit so that I could dictate instructions for him, rather than have him try to read what I wrote.)

I thought that having my staff in the room with me during the office visit allowed for a more relaxed office visit, even though it was expensive to hire more staff. I calculated that having the extra staff actually was cost-effective, because I was then able to see more patients each day, not being bogged down with dictations, and it was less expensive than paying a transcriptionist to type my lengthy, thorough, reports. This was much preferred, rather than the patients or I rushing, talking faster, or they getting undressed and on the exam table more quickly, or I asking them to give one-word answers. But that said, I never objected to short-talking patients who gave only one-word answers anyway. They helped to keep me on time. When the system worked, it was like hitting a homer. It felt good. But its difficulty occurred when a nurse did not show up on a given day or when a nurse was pulled away to cover for another staff member who had not come in that day. For a while, especially during the last year in practice, when we had significant nurse turnover, at least in part related to their not receiving raises and naturally quitting, there was at least one staff member missing every day. When that happened, the buck stopped with me. I had to do all my job and the nurse's job. As one may expect, those days each felt like a week.

No More, Please

I could usually stay reasonably on time in the office unless I heard one of the phrases that most physicians do not want to hear a patient say when they are running late: "Doc, just one more thing ..." This was especially disquieting when I thought that I was done with the visit and ready to move onto the next patient. The day just got longer. I usually knew who my short and long talkers were, where I could catch up time, and where I would fall behind. I knew that I would be in trouble for the day when I had several of what I called my three and four hitters — long talkers with extensive medical problems, analogous to the power hitters in baseball — who would require even more time than usual. I tried to plan accordingly.

God forbid if any patients wanted to share with me some of their hobbies, photographs they had taken, or pictures they had painted, or if they wanted to tell me good jokes or stories that they had just heard. I wanted to see what they wanted to show me or listen to what they wanted to tell me. I considered many of my patients to be my friends and I looked forward to sharing some of their successes with them — as long as I kept an eye on the clock.

I was not so concerned with time management before I went into the practice of medicine. But it became a necessity just to survive the day, once in practice. Intense micromanagement of time became my bad habit, with every second of every day being calculated. It even happened outside the office. I felt like I had a running clock in my head. If, for example, I was talking with a friend, I would know when we had been talking for twenty minutes, even without looking at my watch. Then I would feel like I needed to end the conversation.

At night, when I finally made it home, I enjoyed spending time with my wife and children. I believe that my kids needed my wife and me more and more as they grew older. Changing a diaper, even a diarrhea-filled one, or having a kid spit pureed spinach in my face was easier than trying to help them to resolve their teenage issues. I had no extra energy or patience at night to talk on the phone to a faraway friend or family member to maintain relationships, because I had been talking to people all day. Thus many personal relationships with people whom I truly loved and enjoyed were limited or lost.

Every Second Counts

From 2004 to 2007 at the DEC, patient hours usually began at 7:30 a.m. and ended at 4:00 p.m. I took only twenty minutes for lunch. I even calculated what I would eat for lunch. For example, it was faster to eat pizza or a sandwich than a salad, which took longer because more chewing was involved. Sometimes, during the twenty lunch minutes, I had to decide whether I should actually eat lunch, go to the bathroom, do some urgent paperwork left over from the morning, or talk with the drug representative who had brought in the lunch that day. Sometimes I had to do all of the above. Thus I had a bizarre thought that I should move my desk into the bathroom, so that I could sit on the toilet while I ate with my left hand, did paperwork with my right hand, and talked with the pharmaceutical rep in front of me. That is what the stress of time management can do to one's thought process.

I Could Stay On Time If Only ...

I scheduled twenty-minute office visits and never double-booked, concerned that, if all the patients came, it would be uncomfortable for me, knowing that some patients would be waiting too long, and uncomfortable for them, actually waiting. I counted on the scheduled patients to come. To try to ensure that the patients came, as I could only generate revenue to pay our office expenses when patients were seen in the office, we called all our patients the night or day before to remind them of their office visits the next day. With that, our no show rate was only ten per cent. I used to think that we should sell office visit tickets, much like tickets to a ball game, i.e., whether the person showed up or not, the game would still go on and the players (us) would still get paid. Finally, by the twelfth hour of work, usually with limited breaks, I would admit, "I've had it." I mean, I like playing basketball too, but, after a few hours I would fatigue and — "I've had it."

The major challenge each day was not seeing the scheduled patients and solving their problems; it was trying to do so while multitasking, dealing with all the interruptions and the unexpected, unscheduled "stuff" that occurred all day every day. Examples: Phone calls would come from patients who were either acutely ill or had excessively high or low blood sugars. Doctors would call and need to speak with me ASAP because their patients were in their offices at the time. Phone calls would come from ER physicians treating my patients. I would be filling out insurance preauthorization forms. I would have to get on the phone with insurance personnel if my staff was not able to get an insurance company to approve the urgent test I needed. There were times when I needed to use two phones at once, like a stockbroker.

As a necessity, I became very adept at multitasking, quickly evaluating problems, and making rapid fire decisions. I tried to stick to my motto: "One day, one patient, one problem at a time," but sometimes the problems came in faster than was comfortable for me and I felt like I was in a M*A*S*H unit. Other times I felt like the entertainer on the old *Ed Sullivan Show* who tried to balance spinning plates on more and more sticks without letting them fall, carefully adding more and more plates. However, if one of my plates fell, it would generally mean that something more than a broken dish had occurred. It would mean that something had gone wrong with one of the patients, something that I was desperately trying to avoid.

Single Tasking, A Novel Idea

I was always envious of other professionals, like airline pilots, who had very responsible jobs, but were able to focus on just one task at a time. I could not imagine a pilot receiving a phone call from a passenger in the back of the plane complaining about not getting or liking the snack, or having a tummy ache, or all the bathrooms being occupied. Nor did I think that a pilot would be interrupted just because two passengers got into a conflict. Would the pilot be like my dad driving us kids on long car trips? "I'll stop this plane right here if you guys don't cut it out!" There is a good reason why pilots sit virtually uninterrupted behind closed doors. They must concentrate on only one task, because their loss of either focus or concentration could be fatal to hundreds. It is also no wonder that surgeons are happiest when they are in the operating room (OR). They are protected from outside interference and can focus and concentrate on the task at hand. They do not want any interruption that might make them say the word you never want to hear a surgeon say while operating on a patient: "Oops!"

In retrospect, I think the most pleasant days in the office were during snowstorms, when few patients showed up. It interested me that the ones who did come in were typically those whom I least expected to show up, the seniors. During those wintry days, I had more time to spend with the patients that did come in and there were many fewer phone calls and interruptions. The only problem with those days was financial. One particularly snowy February we lost tens of thousands of dollars because of patient cancellations and no shows.

After Office Hours

Before I moved my practice to the DEC, when patient office hours were over at 3:30 p.m., I would help my nurses, then go to the hospital to check my inpatients or do a consultation for a referring physician. At the DEC, after 4:00 p.m., I would resolve outstanding issues with my nurses, so that they could go home on time, by 4:30. Next, I would call back all the physicians who needed to talk to me that day by 5:00 p.m., before their offices closed. Then I would discuss challenging cases with my nurse practitioner or junior partner so that they could go home by 5:30 or 6:00 p.m. Last, I would settle into my chair for the next one or two hours to review all the papers that had come in that day, such as dictations, doctors' correspondence, and patient labs or imaging studies. If any study was abnormal, which was the case most of the time, given the kinds of patients I was treating, I would review the chart to figure out what the problem was and how to fix it. Sometimes I would call the patient myself, right away, especially if I thought that the matter was urgent. Otherwise, I would write instructions for my nurses to call the patient the next day with my recommendations. If all went well, I could be done with the paperwork by around 7:30 p.m., and then crawl home.

There were times when I just could not get all the paperwork done while still at the office, too tired to finish. Therefore, I packed up my papers in a big gym bag, as heavy as it may be, and schlepped it home to finish the work there, so that I would not fall behind for the next day. I would eat dinner, then sit at the kitchen table and finish the work, rationalizing that at least I was home, around my wife and kids, and so could continue to be involved in their lives. When I finally went to sleep, I would pray that the beeper would not go off overnight — I was on call 24/7 when I was in town — and that I could get my full eight hours of sleep, uninterrupted, and feel refreshed the next morning to repeat the cycle all over again. I know that these hours are not unique to physicians. Marty Nemko, citing Zogby/MSN, mentioned in the September 21, 2007, *U.S. News and World Report* that one third of people making more than $100,000 per year work more than fifty hours per week.

There was a Greek mythological king named Sisyphus who was condemned by Zeus for all eternity to roll a rock up a hill only to have it roll back down when it got to the top. Then he had to roll it back up again, and again, and again, and again ...

I could certainly relate to poor old Sisyphus. But who really condemned me? Was it I myself or was it a consequence of the medical system that drove physicians without procedures to see more patients each day, to try to keep up with our ever decreasing reimbursements and ever increasing expenses?

The Psycho in Right Field

I tried never to miss any of my kids' high school baseball or softball games. If they were playing, I was there. So as not to fall behind in my work, I would back up my SUV near right field and sit in my trunk, with the hatch open facing the field, reviewing papers between innings. I felt like a psycho sitting out there, but I would have felt even worse if I had missed their games, and I felt even worse than that when I had to drive back to the office later some nights to complete the work. In some respects it was good for me to sit far away from the action, since I, like many parents, could easily get caught up in the competition of the game, and say things to the umpires and the opponents that I might later regret.

There Are No Paperwork Elves

Because of the voluminous papers that came in each day, I had a difficult time taking a day off. Believe me; it was not because I did not need to or want to. I know full well what they say about martyrs, "They *were* good people." If I missed a day of paperwork, it would accumulate and there would be double the amount to do the next day. I was also concerned that I could miss a significant abnormal lab test that would need my attention and assessment that day. There were no paperwork elves, who would sneak into the office at night to complete whatever work I did not get done the day before so that, when I walked into the office the next morning, all the work would be done.

A few months before my practice closed, I took a day off to show my mother-in-law, who was in visiting from Chicago, the Thousand Islands, a geographical wonderland in the St. Lawrence River between northern New York State and Ontario. Before we left that morning, I stopped by the office to deal with any urgent issues. Then I calculated how long it would take to drive to the islands and back, grab some lunch, go on a boat tour, and still be back that night in time to do the paperwork that would have accumulated that day.

Even when I had a day off, I would always plan on coming into the office, much to the dismay of my staff, who

would say, "What are you doing here. It's your day off." I
could never comfortably have a full day off without paying
the price of either going in or falling behind. Worse than that,
if I was out of the office for a week, either on vacation or at a
medical education seminar, the amount of paperwork that
would accumulate was sick, which actually made me sick.

To the chagrin of my wife and kids, we always came
back from our vacations two days early so that I could do the
accumulated paperwork. It would take several days on vacation
to catch up on sleep, decompress, and rejuvenate from being
at work. By then I would have started having bad dreams about
going back to work, the most predominant being that I was
late seeing patients in the office and patients were crowding
in the waiting room, which really was my major stressor each
working day. I would also feel angst about returning to work
and finding the build-up of papers. Walking back into the
office after time off was truly difficult, because hundreds of
charts were not only all over my desk and bookshelves but
also on the floor. Anticipating then actually seeing the work
that had accrued while I was gone was always a most demoralizing moment. All this made me consider that any time off
might be not even be worth it.

Dedication of Foolishness?

What made doing the paperwork even more distressing was
that, after about five days off, I would sit at my desk for fifteen to twenty hours over the following two days just on this
task, so that I could have all the papers reviewed and be ready
to start fresh the following Monday. To the dismay of our
business manager, I could not bill anyone for this time spent,
which is called, in the business vernacular, "uncompensated
time." How many lawyers, accountants, or other professionals
would sit there unpaid like that?

Some physicians started charging patients administrative fees to do paperwork on patients' behalf, even when the
patients were not physically present in the office, because paperwork takes nurses' and physicians' time. These physicians
would argue that medicine is indeed a business, and that, given

the increasing amount of paperwork that needs to be done now, compared with years ago, this makes good business sense (cents?). As Linda Zespy reported in "Should You Charge for It?" in the November/December 2004 online issue of *Physicians Practice* at <www.physicianspractice.com/index/fuseaction/ articles.details/articleID/598.htm>, thirty-three per cent of established M.D.s in 2004 spent seven to ten hours per week and another twelve per cent spent eleven to fourteen hours per week doing paperwork, compared with four hours per week when they first went into practice. Their fees were between $5 and $50 per instance, depending on the type and amount of paperwork that needed to be done.

But, not surprisingly, these new fees have not been well received by patients. Although people expect to pay lawyers, accountants, and even plumbers, who get paid just for driving to your home, patients resent such charges from their physicians. Some patients have left physician practices because of this. Although I considered charging administrative fees, I did not think that the few thousand extra dollars that they might generate would be worth the aggravation of patients complaining about them, not to mention my trying to collect the money.

My Preference is Water Torture

Making a lot of money was definitely not why I became a doctor — if it had been I would not have chosen endocrinology. But I did have bills to pay. Those two days of uncompensated time hurt more than so-called "turf toe," because our practice was suffering financially and my excellent, trained staff was quitting, because we could not afford to give them the raises they deserved. It was also torture for me to sit there for that length of time, because I had given up vacation, rest, and rejuvenation, as well as quality time with my family.

This got to the point where I decided that I would not take any prolonged vacations; they just were not worth it. I would rather have suffered the notorious water torture, where a drip of water would bounce off my forehead every second, i.e., do the papers every day even if it meant coming in on a day off, then get hit by a tsunami, i.e., miss several days and try to catch up. To that end, I would limit my time out of the office, even if no patients were scheduled that day. The very thought of returning to Israel, or visiting our own American treasures like our national parks, was out of the question. I felt like I was on a ball and chain, handcuffed to the office, a literal hostage.

The accumulation of papers each day may be more peculiar to non-procedural specialties like endocrinology, internal medicine, or family practice than to other specialties that do not order tests that need constant review. In "How Much Time Do Physicians Spend Providing Care Outside of Office Visits?" in the November 20, 2007, *Annals of Internal Medicine*, Jeffrey Farber *et al.* assessed sixteen geriatricians and determined that these doctors spent an average of 6.7 minutes per patient outside the office for every thirty minutes they spent with that patient in the office. For a geriatrician seeing fourteen patients per day, for thirty minutes at a time, that would be almost eight extra hours of work per week. I was seeing about twenty patients per day at twenty minute intervals. I could do the math to tell you how much extra time I spent per week reviewing papers, but you get the idea.

Some of my radiology friends typically take twelve weeks off per year, that is, on average, one week off per month. They tell me that when they are out of the office their colleagues read the films that come in. When they return to their offices from their vacations, which could be as late as Sunday night before they start reading films again on Monday morning, there are only a few papers to review, or maybe even none. The same is true for my anesthesia friends. When they are gone, they are *gone*. Was I envious? I guess! My wife would sometimes remind me that I could have gone into one of those fields as well, but I would respond that my passion was internal medicine and endocrinology.

If I ever did take a vacation I never wore my watch. Did I know what time it was? Did I care? Does anyone? When I was on vacation I truly did not know or care what time it was. I hoped that each day without wearing a watch would feel longer than twenty-four hours.

Why Not Work Less?

Some of my patients would say, "Doc, you're working too hard. You have to see fewer patients." Kidding, I would reply, "You're right, where do I begin? Let's begin with you." In general, however, it was a legitimate comment. One might indeed say, "Why not work less?" I did not think that it would be feasible for the following four reasons:

First, we were trained and conditioned in medical school and residency to work long and hard hours. If you wanted to be part of the A team, that was how you worked. If I did not work like that, I would feel like I was loafing. In some respects, that became a bad habit. I was also trained from my sports days always to practice and play my hardest. I remember that my basketball coach one day pulled up a chair, sat in it on the sideline, and said, "Men, we're gonna run until I get tired." It took a couple of hours for him, sitting there, to get tired. In the meantime, we ran long and hard.

Second, I had countless patients in my practice. Already I was having difficulty finding time to schedule them even for routine follow-up appointments. I was not willing to perform the patient purge in Syracuse, even as President Bush was performing the military surge in Iraq. I liked ninety-nine per cent of my patients (and that one out of a hundred whom I did not like would never know it, because I treated everyone the same). I did not want any of my patients to leave the practice.

I used to hope that I would not get sick and miss a day in the office. I was no Joe DiMaggio, Lou Gehrig, or Cal Ripken, Jr., but I only missed one day from work — and that was because I thought that it would be wrong to vomit on the patients. If I ever went away, I hoped that my flights were on time, so that I would not get stuck in some faraway city and have to miss time from the office. If that occurred, I did not know how soon I could see the patients who needed to be rescheduled, because the schedule was so filled up for the coming months.

Third, I was not willing to close my practice to new patients, although I did limit them. Not only was it fun and interesting to meet and treat new patients, but also I did not want the referring doctors to have to beg for me to see their patients, especially given the paucity of endocrinologists in our area. Also, it was hard for me to say no to doctors, many of whom were working equally as hard as I. I had deep respect for them. They were my friends and we were on the same team.

I became a victim of my own success. The more time I spent with patients and the better the care they received, the more satisfied they were. Then they would tell their friends or their referring doctors, and more patients would be referred to me. Although my practice continued to grow and to put additional pressure on my time, I continued to try to maintain the strategies that had made me successful, including being kind, caring, compassionate, accessible, communicating well, and always giving the personal touch.

Fourth, I was desperately trying to make up the financial shortfall each month, which otherwise would have to be made up by my employers — and friends — at FPA. The only way to generate revenue was to see patients in the office.

One of my patients did not understand this situation. She had an abnormal bone density and I wanted her to come to the office so that I could better evaluate her case. She lived forty-five minutes from the office, and she did not want to make the drive nor did she want to miss work. I empathized with her, but I also did not think that it was medically sound to deal with this by phone. The case required a significant amount of my time, for which I thought I should be compensated. After all, I have only my skills and services to sell to make a living. She subsequently wrote me a nasty letter letting me know I was just another greedy doctor. That really hurt me, because in the past I had spent a significant amount of time with her and her husband, much of which was not financially compensated, when she was first referred to me for her initial problem, a pituitary tumor.

"R and R" Means "Rest and Reload"

These long hours and this intense commitment to patient care left me little time to rejuvenate, not to mention running errands like getting the few hairs that I have left on my head cut. I also needed time off to stay fresh and sharp, so I could be at my optimal physical and emotional level to deal with the daily challenges that a clinical practice demands. For me, the nights and weekends were not for "R and R," rest and relaxation. Rather, that stood for "rest and reload," because there was so much new information to stay current with in our medical journals, and so many patients' charts to review, so many extra challenges. CPAs may relate to this work intensity by imagining tax season as every day, every month, all year. Lawyers may relate to it by imagining always either preparing for a trial or in one. Athletes may imagine playing their particular sport all year round, every day, with no off-season.

For the thirty years from when I was an undergraduate until I left practice, I was totally focused on being the best doctor I could possibly be, to serve my patients as well as I possibly could. I strongly believe that that is what they deserve, and frankly, it gave me immense pleasure to help them. The enormous amount of time I spent in education and training was well worth it and I would not change anything about that. On the other hand, I felt like I gave up so much of myself to the practice of medicine and commitment to my patients that it was hard to find time to learn or do other things besides being a physician, father, and husband. For me, trying to practice medicine the absolutely right way was all-consuming.

There Is More to Do and Less Time to Do It

In May 2003 Sally Trude stated in *Tracking Report No. 8* of the Center for Studying Health System Change (HSC) that physicians were spending more time in direct patient care: 46.6 hours per week in 2001 compared with 44.7 hours in 1997. But, according to "The Changing Times: Patient Visit Duration with Internists, 1980-1996," a paper given at the 1998 National Research Service Award (NRSA) Trainees' Research Conference by J. Watanabe *et al.*, the amount of time that internal medicine specialists spent with each patient decreased during those sixteen years from twenty-nine to seventeen minutes for new patients and nineteen to sixteen minutes for follow-up visits. The word on the street in 2007 was that the six-minute office visit had become fashionable and was gaining popularity among primary care physicians. Yet according to Trude, thirty-four per cent of physicians did not think that they had enough time to spend with their patients in 2001, compared with twenty-eight per cent in 1997. She also argued that less time with patients adds to physicians' stress, because there are not only more facts to review for patients, especially those with chronic diseases that may require more coordination of services with other treating physicians, but also more ways to test and more options to treat problems. As David Mechanic observed in the *British Medical Journal* (*BMJ*) on August 4, 2001, patients' expectations have also grown higher, given all the medical studies on the best ways to diagnose and treat conditions, as well as a plethora of technological advances.

Patients do not like less time with their physicians either. The study of Chen-Tan Lin *et al.* in the June 11, 2001, *Archives of Internal Medicine*, claimed that the amount of time spent with their physicians during office visits was a major determinant of patients' satisfaction. Less time with patients also reduced preventive care. For example, according to "The Quality of Ambulatory Care Delivered to Children in the United States" by Rita Mangione-Smith *et al.* in the October 11, 2007, *NEJM*, children received the recommended health care forty-seven per cent of the time, and most of those children were white, middle to upper class, and had private insurance.

Less time listening to patients may promote inappropriate referring and prescribing behaviors. Jonas Lundkvist *et al.* concluded in *Family Practice*, volume 19 (2002), that less time spent with patients led to unnecessary antibiotic prescriptions — and higher patient dissatisfaction compared with those physicians who spent more time listening to their patients and prescribed antibiotics less frequently.

Less time with patients may increase the risk of errors and malpractice claims. How could it not? It is only reasonable that when physicians spend less time with patients they have less information to make diagnoses, to institute treatment plans, and to convey to patients. Physicians who take short cuts due to time constraints end up playing the odds, guessing that common things occur commonly, and hoping that they make the correct decisions with limited information. Unfortunately, not all guesses are correct and not all hopes come true.

Less Time With Patients = Increased Errors?

In its classic 1999 report, *To Err is Human: Building a Safer Health System*, the IOM announced that an estimated 44,000 to 98,000 people die each year following preventable medical errors in hospitals, and that these numbers are conservative. A study done in April 2006 by Health Grades, Inc., a leading health care ratings firm, stated that 575,000 people, of which 250,246 were Medicare patients, died in hospitals over a three year period due to preventable medical errors. These deaths do not include those caused by nosocomial (hospital-associated) infections, which are all too common across the country. When I rounded in the hospital before I gave up my hospital practice I regularly saw errors to the point where I once told my wife, half jokingly, "If I get sick, let me die at home instead of getting killed in the hospital."

Medical errors had become so numerous that in August 2007 Medicare decided not to pay for iatrogenic (doctor-caused) errors on hospitalized patients. Certainly one of the ways to reduce the number of malpractice cases, and the associated awards, would be to reduce the number of medical errors. Hospital administrators have also recognized the alarming frequency of these errors. In hopes of eliminating at least some lawsuits, some hospitals forgo charges for treatments that involve preventable serious medical errors, known as "never events."

Compassionate, intelligent people are drawn to the health professions. It is very hard, academically, to be accepted into and to complete these training programs. The root of good medicine is not caring or intelligence, but rather, I believe, at least in part, the time necessary to pay attention to details. It should not be how many patients a doctor can see, but how many can they see *well*. It takes time to take a thorough history. It takes time to do an appropriate physical examination. It takes time to review the lab and imaging tests and then to consider all the pieces of the puzzle or to connect all the dots to solve a patient's riddle, to determine what is really the most accurate diagnosis and the best treatment and follow-up. It takes time to review this information with the patients so that they can understand their problems and help with their treatment.

The Time Spent Was Worth It

There were countless instances in my practice where a problem
was averted or solved because I took extra time with a patient
to discover a problem that was not readily apparent. For example, a diabetic patient with very poorly controlled blood
sugars, despite having been prescribed massive amounts of
insulin, was referred to me. After racking my brain for thirty
or forty minutes with the patient, asking multiple questions,
trying to solve the conundrum of why he was on so much insulin and still had poor glycemia, I finally asked him how long
a bottle of insulin lasted him. He said, "A few months." Given
the amounts of insulin he was taking, a bottle of insulin should
have lasted him only a few days. I then asked him, right then
and there, to draw up insulin into a syringe. He drew up
mostly air! No wonder his blood sugars were high. He was
hardly giving himself any insulin at all, even though he thought
he was giving himself more and more. "Who would've thunk
it?" Once this was discovered, his blood sugars normalized
and he was on only a fraction of the amount of insulin that
had been prescribed to him before he came to my practice.
Taking time with that patient, which allowed me to pay closer
attention to details, enabled me to resolve the issue.

Take My Time, Really?

Since I left practice in October 2007, I have been a consultant
for medical malpractice attorneys doing defense work. Their
initial instructions to me were to take as much time as I needed
with each case that I reviewed to make sure that I knew all its
details and could render my best opinion to either defend or
settle it. After all, thousands to millions of dollars could be at
stake. Some cases took me up to ten hours to review. I am
convinced that the majority of the malpractice cases that I
reviewed could have been avoided if the provider had taken
more time to assess the case properly, and not jumped to the
most common cause of the complaint. For example, chest
pain in a fifty-year-old male is commonly due to coronary
artery disease, but could, as in this case, be symptomatic of a

fatal dissecting aortic aneurysm that the physician had missed. Doctors need time to consider all the possible causes of each patient's symptoms. They should not feel the need to go as quickly as they can, so as to move on to each next case.

I have been there. I knew what it was like to have several cases backed up, with the desire burning to make decisions as quickly as possible, so that I could move on to the next case while I still had energy — and be lucky enough to make it home that night before my family went to sleep. What seems perverse to me in 2009 is that not only am I compensated much better as a medical consultant than I was when actually treating patients in the office, but I can now also take as much time as I need to give my best opinion. Could I take as much time as I needed to solve a case while in clinical practice? That just did not happen, unless it was on my own time, after weekday patient hours or on weekends.

No Time Yet Just to Sit on the Dock

Our medical mentors never suggested, nor should they have, that we take short cuts, spend less time with our patients, or not address all of each patient's concerns at one office visit. Heck, one concern of a patient might be related to another concern, and then to another, and if you only address one and not the others, then the pieces of the puzzle as to what is causing the problems may not be solved. Also, our mentors never told us to stand with our hand on the doorknob while a patient was talking to us. On the contrary, they educated us to set up the exam room so that it was comfortable first for the patients, second for their accompanying family members, and finally for us. To sit and make level eye contact with patients, so that they know that we care about them, to listen intently, and to let patients finish their sentences — that makes all the difference. We have two ears and one mouth for a reason, to do more listening than speaking. Do the patients not deserve all these courtesies? After all, they left their homes or jobs to come to see us — not the other way around — and they waited in our waiting or exam rooms until we were ready to see them. We owe them our full attention for as long as it might take to help them.

Do medical office visits have to be as they have become, so short, impersonal, and abrupt? The patients do not like this state of affairs. The doctors do not like it. Certainly the defense malpractice insurance companies do not like it. It is bad medicine and dangerous. Then why does it persist? There must be a better way.

In the meantime, since I have been out of practice, there has been a lot of time that I have needed to catch up on. I have not set my alarm clock once nor have I worn my watch. I still go to sleep at the same time I did when I was in practice, but I wake up an hour later. I exercise every day for an hour and I now go the actual speed limit while driving. I talk with my faraway friends and family by phone more often and, who knows, maybe one day soon I will even sit on Otis Redding's dock — but probably not until the American health care system is fixed.

Chapter Eleven

Malpractice

The "Scarlet Letter"

OK, I admit it. I was sued for malpractice in 1998. I have a "scarlet letter." There, I said it and I am totally embarrassed about it. You do not have to go looking for my name in the National Practitioner Data Bank, it is out in the open, although, if you do search that database, you will find my name along with many other dedicated, committed, respected, and, respectfully, talented physicians. Being sued was, without question, the lowest point of my professional life and certainly one of the five worst things that have ever happened to me. I still get upset about it, though it happened so many years ago! The pain associated with being sued was immeasurable. From that time forward my professional life would never be the same. I would do anything not to have another malpractice attorney shoot another arrow at the bull's-eye on my back.

The Details of the Case

The allegation was that I and two other doctors missed a diagnosis of pseudotumor cerebri in an unemployed woman on Medicaid whom I was treating for Cushing's disease, a condition wherein the adrenal glands secrete excess amounts of one of its hormones, cortisol. As a last resort to treat her Cushing's disease, she had a bilateral adrenalectomy, initially attempted laparoscopically by the surgeon, but then converted to an open procedure due to internal bleeding.

Almost immediately post-operation, she complained of neck pains and occipital headaches that waxed and waned. The symptoms were positional and the working diagnosis was that she had a musculoskeletal strain. We thought that maybe she had been put into an odd position, either on the OR table or in the recovery room, or maybe she had been injured while being transferred from the stretcher to the operating table or to her bed. There was no concern to us at that time that she had any central nervous system consequence of her surgery, insofar as the operation had been in her abdomen, her pains were worse when she moved her neck, and she had no focal neurological deficits. A CT scan of her brain was also normal.

After she left the hospital, initially feeling better and with fewer symptoms, her headaches returned. I was in contact with her frequently, phoning her nights and weekends to see how she was doing, because she was on my worried list. She lived over an hour away and had limited transportation, otherwise I would have seen her in the office. She was seeing her primary care provider near her home and was also going to physical therapy. Another CT scan of her brain was again normal. Several weeks after the operation she complained of sudden loss of vision. The accurate diagnosis of pseudotumor cerebri, an increase in intracranial pressure not caused by a tumor, was finally made. As it turned out, we diagnosed her with an unusual familial clotting condition. This condition made her more susceptible to blood clots, which occurred in the large veins that drain blood from the brain. These clots caused the increase in intracranial pressure, which put pressure on her eye nerves, which caused her loss of vision. Unfortunately, such clots cannot be seen on routine CT scans. Rather, a special MRI of the intracranial veins, an MRV (magnetic resonance venogram), would have been needed.

We also found that she had been given a diagnosis of pseudotumor cerebri almost fifteen years prior by a neurologist, when she had had the same type of headaches. At her legal deposition, when she was asked why she had not told us about that history, she replied, "I didn't think of it." OUCH! Here we were, doctors, worried about her continued headaches, desperately trying to figure out why she was having them, calling her on the phone, seeing her in the office, unable to come up with the cause — and she had had the answer the whole time. If that patient had been you, wouldn't you have mentioned it to the doctor?

No Good Deed Goes Unpunished

Prior to being sued, I had followed all the advice that had been given to us by a very aggressive malpractice plaintiff's attorney when I was in medical school. Who wouldn't? He scared the pants off us. He had "The Look": black hair combed back with Brylcreem, a very expensive suit, and such tiny glasses that you could not see his eyes. Intimidating? Yes!

I felt like I had developed an excellent rapport with this patient. I had enjoyed caring for her. I spent enormous amounts of time with her and her boyfriend, diagnosing and coming up with a suitable treatment plan for her, given some of the complexities of her case and her limited financial situation. I even had one of my mentors, who had written a textbook on adrenal diseases, see her — in *my* office and free of charge — for a second opinion.

I would treat every patient the same, i.e., like a VIP. She was no exception. I followed all the suggestions given to us by the intimidating malpractice attorney to avoid lawsuits, including developing physician/patient relationships based on caring, compassion, and straightforward communication. I took all the appropriate medical steps to diagnose and treat her Cushing's disease. She admitted to me later that her boyfriend had actually instigated the lawsuit, evidently smelling some easy money. Given all the challenges of the case, including the fact that the company providing my malpractice insurance at that time was going out of business, I begrudgingly accepted settlement rather than fight the case at a jury trial, where, if you lose, you can lose big.

A Jury of My Peers Does Not Exist

Frankly, I would have preferred not to have given consent to settle this case. I would instead have taken it to trial, because I thought that I had met the standard of care, but a jury of my peers does not exist. A jury of my peers would be a jury of other doctors in my specialty. Cases like mine are incredibly complicated, even for physicians trained in the field. The jury, untrained in medical matters, would have heard potentially confusing and conflicting testimony about standards of care from me, the patient, and various expert witnesses. To leave to them the decision as to whether I and the two other defendants had committed malpractice or not would have been very risky. The jury would have had to decide whom to believe, without any clear guidelines on what medically acceptable standards are. They may have let their own natural sympathy for the plaintiff, a blind, poverty-stricken woman, steer their decision. In "Relation between Negligent Adverse Events and the Outcomes of Medical-Malpractice Litigation" in the December 26, 1996, *NEJM*, Troyen Brennan *et al.* concluded that, even when there was no gross malpractice, a jury might still find in favor of the plaintiff if the plaintiff had suffered a significant disability.

The Progressive Policy Institute (PPI), in its February 2005 *Policy Report*, and the AMA, in its June 2007 draft of principles, touted health courts to replace the American malpractice system of deciding whether medical malpractice had occurred and, if it had, what damages should be awarded. Instead of having medical malpractice cases heard in civil courts, there would be a special health court, analogous to workers compensation boards, where a specially trained and qualified judge, without a jury, would determine the standards for malpractice, hear arguments from medical experts hired by the courts, and then, if there was malpractice, determine awards based on a predetermined schedule of economic and non-economic factors set by an independent commission created by Congress. Each health court would publicly report cases settled or adjudicated.

State-level health courts would ideally give injured persons greater access to legal remedies and quicker adjudication of their claims, which in the civil court system might take upwards of five years to resolve. The case in which I was involved did indeed take almost five years to resolve. That was a long five years for me, having that constantly hanging over my head. I suspect that physicians involved in lawsuits are at a greater risk of generating further lawsuits during the time of the ongoing lawsuit, because they are less focused on their current patients and more distracted by the details of the legal case. I can relate. I frequently spaced out over the proceedings of my malpractice case and constantly had to bring myself back.

Health courts may also be less expensive than civil courts in evaluating malpractice cases. According to a Harvard School of Public Health study, "Claims, Errors, and Compensation Payments in Medical Malpractice Litigation" by David Studdert, Michelle Mello, Atul Gawande, *et al.*, in the May 11, 2006, *NEJM*, litigating a claim then cost an average of $52,000, including defense administration and lawyers' contingency fees, or fifty-four per cent of the plaintiff's compensation.

This idea of an administrative replacement for the American malpractice system has been a topic of discussions and writings since the 1990s. The 2005 PPI report noted that many European jurisdictions had already experienced success with such systems. Also in 2005, Senators Michael B. Enzi (R-Wyoming) and Max Baucus (D-Montana) introduced the Fair and Reliable Medical Justice Act (S-1337) as a bill in the 109th Congress. It was reported favorably out of the Senate Health, Education, Labor, and Pensions Committee, but went no further. In 2007, Representatives Jim Cooper (D-Tennessee), Mac Thornberry (R-Texas), and two co-sponsors introduced a similar bill, the Fair and Reliable Medical Justice Act (HR-2497) in the 110th Congress. Meanwhile, Baucus and Enzi reintroduced the Senate version as S-1481. Among other things, these bills would authorize "state demonstration programs to evaluate alternatives to current medical tort litigation." Despite broad bipartisan approval, and the support of several patients' rights groups, as of June 2009 none of them had yet become law. Why not? Big-money lobbyists?

Lessons Learned

Being sued was a real black eye event. My wife, an attorney, tried to console me by telling me, "It's just the cost of doing business," and "You aren't a bad doctor you just had a bad outcome." Although she is an extremely kind, caring person and very sympathetic to what I went through, she is used to arm's-length business relationships with her clients. But as a physician I was deeply involved with all my patient's physical, emotional, and social issues. This patient was no exception. I did not think that I could truly help people to achieve optimal health unless I addressed all the components that make up "health." Like the three-legged stool (which for centuries has been the standard metaphor for the three aspects of medicine: teaching, research, and patient care), if one of the three legs breaks, the stool falls over.

I look back on that case and come up with three main thoughts:

First, I did hundreds of things right for that nice woman, but missed one. If I were taking a test, I might have gotten ninety-nine out of a hundred correct, which, in most classes, would be an A or A+. In fact, to pass some of our certification exams, one only needs to get sixty to seventy per cent correct. But this event was no test. When it comes to being a doctor and treating patients in the real world, 99/100, 999/1000, or even 9999/10,000 is just not good enough.

People understand that doctors are human. Patients certainly want and deserve the human elements of kindness, compassion, and empathy. People also understand and accept that errors will be made — as long as those errors are not on them. If we do miss one, and if we are sued, then it may feel like all the successes that we achieved in the past for that person and all our other patients have been negated. Any physician who is asked to recall the details of her/his last great case may have a hard time remembering the facts. But ask physicians to recall details of any case that went bad and they will be able to recite those details as if it all happened yesterday.

I would have traded all my *Best Doctors* awards not to have had the lawsuit. Unfortunately, a physician cannot accumulate points for good care. but just lose points for missed care. The best a doctor could do, if one were to keep score, would be a 0-0 game. But being a doctor is no game. The stakes are much higher. One may feel terrible about striking out in the bottom of the ninth inning with the tying run on third, or about missing both the game-tying and the game-winning foul shots with no time left on the clock, but no one will sue you for those shortcomings. As a physician desperately trying to make my patients' health better, I would say, if everything had gone well at the end of each day, "no morbidity, no mortality, no lawsuits," just like a baseball announcer would say, "no runs, no hits, no errors" at the end of a perfect game.

Second, because of the potential for both the patient's and the doctor's pain and suffering as a consequence of a missed diagnosis, doctors may cope by ordering more tests than are needed or by practicing medicine even more defensively than is practical. Ask doctors what worries them most about practicing medicine. Some will say being sued, especially those who have been sued already and know first-hand the pain associated with the process. After a lawsuit, some may feel angry, depressed, cynical, anxious, or even paranoid about their patients, not to mention tainted, as if they were bad doctors. Their self-esteem may take a hit, especially because, as Thomas Hobbs and Gregory Gable argued in "Coping with Litigation Stress" in the January 1998 *PND*, doctors' identity is defined by their work. Many physicians feel regret, because the thought that they may ever have hurt someone is incongruous with why they went into medicine in the first place. One of the rules of Hippocrates, from his *Epidemics*, is if you cannot cure a disease, then at least do not make it worse, or if you cannot do good, then at least do no harm. From the loose Latin translation of this idea, *primum non nocere*, comes the standard Hippocratic motto in English, "First, do no harm."

Many of us already practice defensive medicine as a necessity. Doctors hate to miss diagnoses and give wrong treatments. I am sure that patients hate it even more. We, the physicians, are in the proverbial pickle. We order tests to make sure that we do not miss any diagnoses, but ordering tests also raises the amount of spending on health care, which also hurts the patient by increasing insurance premiums. I hate to think that some physicians may order unnecessary tests just to profit from them.

"Physicians' Personal Malpractice Experiences are not

Related to Defensive Clinical Practices," a study by Peter Glass-
man, John Rolph, *et al.*, in the Summer 1996 issue of the *Journal
of Health Politics, Policy and Law*, concluded that doctors did not
change their practice styles because of their encounters with the
malpractice system. I suspect that those physicians surveyed
were already practicing defensively, as was I, prior to my lawsuit. But after I was sued I had no hesitations. If I thought of
a test, I ordered it. If I thought a patient needed a second
opinion, I offered it. I was not going to go through that torture again if I could help it.

Third, it is good to use judgment as long as the judgment
is right. Countless times I made a decision, held my breath,
and sweated it out, hoping that all was right with the patient.

Good Judgment is Good

One example that stands out was when I was in my second
year of residency. An elderly woman came into the ER late at
night complaining of abdominal pain. The ER doctor thought
that she had constipation and was treating her with cathartics
hoping to "get her out of the ER ASAP."

Her complaints continued. I was called to see her
around 1:00 a.m. to finish "the cleanout." The story did not
add up. She was not a "frequent flyer" to the ER, i.e., she did
not come often to the ER with nebulous complaints and she
did not seem like a chronic complainer. Her abdominal x-ray
did not show that she was "FOS" ("full of shit"). In short,
there was nothing to clean out. Her abdominal pain was out
of proportion to physical findings, which was something that
I had been told to pay attention to when I did my surgical
clerkship during my third year of medical school. She also had
a subtle abnormality in one of the blood tests, a slightly elevated anion gap. This suggested that she was producing acids
in her body more quickly than her body could buffer them.

I was now faced with a judgment: either continue the
cleanout plan as suggested by the ER attending physician, and
hope that she got better, or risk waking a potentially irate sur-

geon in the middle of the night with my concern that a significant intra-abdominal problem was present. I chose the latter. The woman was taken to the OR a couple of hours after I called the surgeon. I went with her to observe the consequences of my decision. She turned out to have "dead gut," a lack of blood flow to her small bowel, which, if it had gone undiagnosed any longer, would have meant her death and maybe a lawsuit for me for misdiagnosis. Indeed the surgeon's mottos held true that night: "When in doubt, cut it out." — "The only thing between the surgeon and the diagnosis is the skin."

I am not aware of any doctor being sued for getting a consultation or ordering a test, only for not doing either. But if you just once come to a wrong conclusion without a second opinion, or if you just once fail to order a test that could confirm the clinical impression, then be prepared to meet the "I'm-only-protecting-the-patient-from-you-bad-doctors" lawyer who, by the way, is gracious enough to work for a one-third contingency fee.

Given that the woman who sued me was on Medicaid throughout her many years as my patient, I likely made only about $100 from her, even though I put all my physical and emotional energy into trying to help her, in countless hours of caring for her and worrying about her condition. Her malpractice attorney, on the other hand, made six figures settling her case. Is that justice? You tell me.

Scars Are Permanent

I do not begrudge malpractice attorneys, but I do admit continuing to feel rage and disgust at the attorney who sued me when I hear his voice on the radio or see his face on his obnoxious TV advertisements, even though it had been years since my case was adjudicated. For better or worse, I, like many sued physicians, took it very personally. Sometimes I still feel that he went after me. Other times I suspect that he treated the lawsuit against me as just another case and probably did not care who the physician was whom he was suing.

I was also repulsed that his wife was a pediatrician. I felt that he should not be suing doctors, because he was married to one.

I also resented how much money this lawyer made by representing the woman who sued me. I thought that he did not really care about the person he was representing, other than that she could be worth a lot of money to him. If she had been worth less to him monetarily, he likely would not have cared about her injuries at all. Yet on the other hand, speaking more broadly, lawyers may actually be an ironic roadblock to some malpractice cases. They tend to be most interested in egregious cases where large awards are possible; but they tend to turn down cases with little monetary value, even if there was real negligence or malpractice that left patients with true injuries, but small damages, little recourse.

Malpractice Issues Clarified

Malpractice attorneys are an easy target for us physicians. On them we focus our disapproval of the malpractice judicial system and the significant costs that it encumbers. Lawyers are the face on the problem. Physicians feel that there is an over-abundance of frivolous lawsuits, i.e., those without evidence of substandard care or of injury related to treatment. Such lawsuits are incredibly upsetting and stressful for physicians. They are also expensive, because malpractice insurance carriers may then impose surcharges on physicians' premiums.

Studdert, Mello, Gawande, *et al.*, reported in their 2006 *NEJM* article that only twenty-eight per cent of frivolous claims received payment compared with seventy-three per cent paid for claims that actually involved errors. Average payments for non-error cases amounted to two thirds of the payments for error cases. This Harvard study concluded that the malpractice system gets it right about three fourths of the time. Doctors who are sued for frivolous reasons fantasize about countersuing attorneys whose original lawsuits dragged them through the mud. But it is difficult, expensive, and time-consuming to find lawyers willing to sue other lawyers. So most doctors just put the horrible experience behind them and get on with their lives.

But to be fair, lawyers, even those who bring frivolous lawsuits hoping to "win the lottery," are not the only problem with the malpractice system. Physicians' significant costs for malpractice premiums are going up, but not because there are too many malpractice attorneys or malpractice cases. According to the April 2005 Public Citizen Congress Watch report, "Medical Malpractice Payout Trends, 1991-2004," the number of payouts to patients was flat, the number of jury verdicts increased by only 1.2 per cent per year, but the total amount of payments doubled from 2.1 billion to 4.2 billion dollars during those fourteen years, even though the number of payments equal to or greater than one million dollars, adjusted for inflation, decreased fifty-six per cent. In March 2008 the Insurance Information Institute (III) reported on its Web site <www.iii. org> that both Gen Re, a reinsurer of malpractice companies, and Aon, an insurance broker, had verified that while the number of malpractice claims were either stabilizing or decreasing, the associated costs and the amounts of awards were increasing.

"Medical Malpractice Payout Trends, 1991-2004" reported that eighty-three per cent of doctors had no malpractice payouts since 1990, when the National Practitioner Data Bank <www.npdb-hipdb.hrsa.gov/npdb.html> was established. Yet, Angela M. Dodge and Steven F. Fitzer estimated in *When Good Doctors Get Sued: A Guide for Defendant Physicians Involved in Malpractice Lawsuits* (2001) that between fifty and sixty-five per cent of physicians get sued at least once in their careers; i.e., there is at least a 50/50 chance that any given physician will be sued while practicing medicine in America. The March 2005 *PND* reported that 5600 doctors had been sued in Pennsylvania alone from May 2002 to November 2004, an average of six doctors a day for thirty months. Therefore, a doctor who has not yet been sued either is just plain lucky or has not been in practice long enough. Plenty of good doctors, who did not do anything wrong, still get sued. It is no wonder that doctors are anxious, worried, or even paranoid about being sued, es-

pecially when they hear their colleagues' stories about the associated aggravation, even when there is no merit in the cases.

More Myths Debunked

Again according to "Medical Malpractice Payout Trends, 1991-
2004," five and a half per cent of all the doctors were responsible for 57.3 per cent of all the payouts to patients and only a
fraction of the doctors who were repeat offenders were disciplined by their state boards. For example, only 32.5 per cent
of physicians who have had ten or more malpractice cases had
been so disciplined. In my state, New York, according to a
November 2007 report, "A Self-Inflicted 'Crisis': New York's
Medical Malpractice Insurance Troubles Caused By Flawed
State Rate Setting and Raid on Rainy Day Fund," 6186 doctors
made two or more malpractice payouts between 1990 and 2006.
In other words, just 7.7 per cent of all New York doctors accounted for seventy-one per cent of all malpractice payouts.

According to Tom Baker in *The Medical Malpractice
Myth* (2005), the dramatic increase in malpractice premiums
has not been due to more and more injured patients suing
their physicians. Quite the contrary. In fact, Dan Groszkru-
ger's article, "Physician-Patient Dialogue" at the Cooperative
of American Physicians / Mutual Protection Trust Web site
<www.cap-mpt.com>, mentioned that the preponderance of
studies has confirmed the reluctance of most patients to sue
their doctors. Nor has this rise been due to runaway juries,
but rather to the economic cycles and competitive nature of
the medical malpractice insurance industry. Sometimes even
outside influences have played their parts. On March 4, 2008,
James T. Mulder reported in the Syracuse *Post-Standard* that,
in order to replenish malpractice insurance companies' reserves, which had been depleted when New York Governor
George Pataki transferred 691 million of their dollars into the
state's general fund, State Insurance Commissioner Eric R.
Dinallo was threatening a $50,000 malpractice premium sur-
charge, beyond the fourteen per cent that premiums had in-

creased since the previous July.

Regardless of why there are increases in malpractice premiums, there have been concerns that states without either tort reforms or caps on non-economic damages have been losing physicians. Financial analyst David Matsa of Northwestern University partially debunked that theory in his June 20, 2006, article on the Social Science Research Network Web site <www.ssrn.com>. He argued that, while there was a twelve per cent increase in the number of rural physicians from 1970 to 2000 in states with caps, there was no appreciable change in the overall supply of physicians in those states. Mark Pauly, Christy Thompson, *et al.*, reported in "Who Pays? The Incidence of High Malpractice Premiums" in the 2006 *Forum for Health Economics and Policy* that physicians' net incomes did not decline between 1994 and 2002, despite significant increases in malpractice premiums.

More Lessons Learned

Despite some encouraging statistics, the concern about malpractice puts a significant strain on physicians. I know that people my age are largely a sandwich generation, because many of us are sandwiched between caring for our elderly parents while still caring for our children. As doctors, we are also sandwiched between, on one side, ordering tests to make diagnoses, to ensure that we do not miss anything, and, on the other side, the health insurance companies' obstructions that prevent us from obtaining these studies. Because their goals are financial — money matters most — we must endure preauthorizations, sitting endlessly on the phone waiting for non-medical people to reject the ordered tests, etc.! Catch-22? Between a rock and a hard place? Call it what you like, but there we are and it is totally unpleasant.

After the lawsuit I turned my obsessive-compulsive behavior up a notch, which I had not thought was possible. I became even more meticulous about reviewing patient charts, both in the exam room and at my home at night and on weekends.

I learned a lot from being sued, including that the answer to a patient problem is frequently hidden in the patient chart.

The woman who sued me filled out a form when we first met. In retrospect, that was the answer to her case. She wrote, "cerbral edma" [sic]. Given all the other complicated things that were going on with her at our initial visit — a full hour, during which I evaluated the signs and symptoms associated with her Cushing's disease, the tests that had been done to date, the treatments for her out-of-control blood pressure and blood sugars, and some of the significant emotional issues that frequently accompany this condition — I did not spend any time on trying to figure out what "cerbral edma" meant. In fact, it meant "cerebral edema," and was due to pseudotumor cerebri.

I also learned that I could never put my guard down. Even though I may see a patient in the ER complaining of routine chest pain likely due to coronary artery disease, I always keep my guard up and go to the obvious diagnosis last, because that makes me consider other sneaky possibilities, like a pulmonary embolus or a dissecting aortic aneurysm. In medical lingo, this is called going through a differential diagnosis list. I learned that even though something may look like a horse, smell like a horse, and walk like a horse, it could still be a zebra. In doctor jargon, "zebra" means an unusual, rare diagnosis. As I learned from reviewing numerous malpractice case records, undiagnosed zebras with bad outcomes often get sued and usually result in payouts.

Many of us physicians voluntarily take a six-or-seven-hour home tutorial every two years, sponsored by our medical liability companies, on ways to avoid malpractice. The incentive to take the course is receiving a five per cent discount on malpractice premiums.

Compared with horror movies like *The Shining*, *The Exorcist*, or *The Omen*, the information in this course is much scarier. All prospective medical students should learn it before they decide whether to go to medical school, so that they may know what the stakes are before committing to the enormous sacrifices and risks that would be ahead of them. Do you think that many of them would still choose to attend medical school, if they really knew first-hand the risks of just being good-natured? Would it be worth so much of their time, money, and self-sacrifice to be involved in a game where one loss could outweigh all their victories? Maybe it is just too dangerous to be a doctor.

What is an Error Anyway?

There are countless ways for clinicians, nurses, and other health care professionals to make errors. I suspect that, if a group of us sat around a table and tried to come up with all the ways, we would still miss some. What is an error? One might think that the answer would be obvious. In many situations it is, such as operating on the wrong extremity, missing breast cancer on a mammogram, or giving a medication to a patient with a known allergy to that medication. However, a study published by Nancy Elder, Harini Pallerla, and Saundra Regan in the December 8, 2006, issue of *BMC Family Practice*, concluded that no general agreement exists among physicians about what constitutes an error.

There are at least twenty-five different definitions of "medical error" in the literature. Elder, Pallerla, and Regan surveyed 285 family practitioners and asked them to judge five common scenarios. All agreed that overlooking an abnormal lab was wrong. Eighty-seven per cent thought that performing the wrong test and not following up an abnormal test were errors. Sixty-two per cent thought it was an error not to have an imaging study result available during a patient visit. Forty-seven per cent thought it was an error to break a blood tube. Medical life, like life in general, is certainly all shades of gray.

It's OK to Say I'm Sorry

How physicians respond to mistakes is yet another question. Thomas Gallagher, Amy Waterman, *et al.*, stated in the *Ar-*

chives of Internal Medicine, August 14-28, 2006, that ninety-eight per cent of about 1650 American and Canadian physicians surveyed thought that honesty was the best policy and recommended disclosing serious errors to patients.

Grena G. Porto is a nationally recognized expert in risk management and patient safety, founder of QRS Healthcare Consulting, and former Senior Director of Clinical Consulting for Voluntary Hospitals of America (VHA), an alliance of 2200 community-based hospitals. She believes that patients will forgive physicians for mistakes if the physicians disclose and discuss their errors promptly, fully, sincerely, compassionately, and without any spin, or dancing around the issue. Also, when appropriate, a patient may desire an apology without the physician necessarily going overboard. Just a simple "I'm sorry this complication has occurred" or "I'm sorry it turned out this way" may suffice.

Patients interviewed on this topic have consistently stated that physicians have no idea how far a "sorry" will go. Although doctors may feel upset, guilty, alone, have loss of self-esteem, and are sometimes unsure where to go to seek emotional support to help them deal with errors, it remains generally true that, by pulling themselves together and showing contrition, they are less likely to get sued.

Gallagher and Waterman led another team in an earlier study, published in *JAMA*, February 26, 2003, which discussed physicians' concerns that their apologies to patients might create legal liabilities. By 2007, to alleviate such concerns, about thirty states had enacted "I'm sorry" laws to forbid patients from using their physicians' apologies for medical mistakes against the physicians in court. Nevertheless, as Tom Delbanco and Sigall Bell described in "Guilty, Afraid, and Alone: Struggling with Medical Error" in the October 25, 2007, *NEJM*, frightened physicians continue to struggle with conflicting personal principles, moral and professional ethics, and institutional policies.

Patients Have Responsibilities Too

I do not believe that all the responsibility for patient care should fall on the physician. Patients, who are also my teammates, should also have responsibilities. For example, doctors are responsible when we order tests or refer patients to other physicians for consultation, and the patients do not go. If they do not go, we are supposed to contact them, find out why not, and then spend more of our time and limited resources to send them certified letters if we cannot reach them by phone, asking them to contact us so that we can reschedule their appointments. We assume full liability for their behaviors. How could that be right?

We also assume full liability, without compensation, for phone calls from patients during or after hours. Who thought of that system? Lawyers and accountants do not play by those rules. A patient can call us anytime, day or night, for free, and we had better document the interaction. A lawyer friend of mine once said, "If it was not documented, then it was not done." But just because it was documented does not mean that it *was* done, which might especially be true in newly installed EMR systems. For example, these EMRs can easily insert information into an office visit note, thus upgrading the code, so that the provider may get paid more for that office visit. Any notes that physicians generate are legal documents. However, unlike in the court system, where legal documents are also generated, we do not have stenographers to produce these legal papers in our exam rooms and certainly not in our homes when we take middle-of-the-night phone calls.

If patients called me in the middle of the night, I usually thought that they were either crazy or really sick, and sometimes it was hard to tell the difference. At 3:00 a.m. one night, after I had just gotten home from the hospital and fallen asleep, a young woman called to tell me that she had hypothyroidism and was cold. Understand that among the main symptoms of hypothyroidism is cold intolerance, but it is certainly not a medical emergency necessitating a 3:00 a.m. phone call. At that time of night, associated with significant sleep deprivation, I usually forget all the approved Dale Carnegie techniques for winning friends and influencing people. So I asked her, "Are you crazy?" She promptly hung up on me, which was a sure sign that she was not nuts. A crazy person would stay on the phone just being happy to have someone to talk with, even if I were belligerent. I quickly called her back, apologized for my comment, and determined that what she meant by "being cold" was that she was having chills and rigors. I recalled Riddle Solving 101. I sent her to the ER, where she was diagnosed with pyelonephritis, a severe infection of her kidney. She was treated appropriately and she did fine.

It is obvious that we live in a litigious society. When people feel wronged we much prefer them to seek compensation civilly through the courts than to take matters into their own hands — like shooting someone. Doctors are sometimes murdered. In 1987, Dr. Herbert Lourie, one of Syracuse's most esteemed neurosurgeons, was shot and killed at his home, point blank, by a disgruntled relative of one of his patients. When I was involved with my lawsuit, knowing that the plaintiff's boyfriend was disgruntled and, so I believed, unstable, I was cautious before going outside each morning. Being sued certainly trumps being shot, but I would not choose either.

After I was sued, anytime I saw a piece of paper with what was, or appeared to be, an attorney's letterhead, I was like a Pavlov dog. It would give me an immediate fight or flight response. I still have not gotten over this feeling of fight or flight whenever I see a lawyer's name at the top of a page — even though I am long out of private practice.

Standard of Care

As a reviewer of malpractice cases, I am asked to judge if the provider who is being sued has met the community's standard of care. The standard of care, defined in legal terms, is the level at which the average, prudent provider in a given community would practice. It is how similarly qualified practitioners would have managed patients' care under the same or similar circumstances. But medicine is not all science. There is no guideline, no sufficiently defined standard of care, nor enough evidence-based medicine to cover every scenario that could possibly happen. A large part of what physicians do is art: the art of diagnosis, the art of judgment, the art of dealing with people, the art of coping with the unfamiliar.

For example, I reviewed the case of an elderly male patient who had coronary artery disease, atrial fibrillation, and renal insufficiency. He called his primary care doctor's office one day, complaining of new onset lower extremity swelling, but no shortness of breath or chest pain. A nurse took the patient's phone call and communicated the findings to the doctor, who prescribed a diuretic, Lasix, to be taken each day. Unfortunately, the only documentation of that phone call was that the Lasix prescription had been called into the pharmacy. No other details of the history or follow-up were written down.

This poor documentation certainly did not meet the standard of care, or any standard of documentation, but a second aspect of the situation was compelling to me with regard to determining a standard of care. Should the doctor have offered the patient an office visit before giving him Lasix, especially with his new symptom in the context of advanced and already known medical problems? What kind of follow-up plans should have been made once he started taking Lasix?

Three weeks after the patient started taking Lasix, he died. His wife thus inferred that Lasix had caused her husband's death and was suing the provider for prescribing this medication. Determining cause and effect is one of the most difficult challenges a physician can have. Did Lasix cause his death? Did the diuretic cause some electrolyte disturbance and a subsequent cardiac arrhythmia? Or did he die because of an underlying condition that made him need a medication like Lasix in the first place, perhaps degenerative kidney disease or undiagnosed heart failure. Or maybe he died for completely unrelated reasons, perhaps a clot in his lung. Regardless of these possibilities, what should have been the standard of care been in treating this case?

I asked the other board-certified internist and the family

practitioner, who both also review medical malpractice cases for the same company. I received two different answers — both different from what I would have done.

I would have insisted that the patient be seen in my office, or go to the ER, before I prescribed Lasix. "Lebowitz's Rule # 1," which has never failed me, is to err always on the side of safety. Why chance danger? What could have been safer than to see the patient and determine what was wrong before prescribing the medication, especially given the multitude of possible reasons for the swelling? It could have been due to a benign cause, like eating too much salt or sitting in a chair too long, or to something significant, like heart, liver, or kidney failure.

Also, I would have wanted a follow-up appointment and lab tests soon after starting Lasix, because that drug could adversely affect potassium and calcium levels as well as renal function, which could subsequently affect his other medications, such as the digoxin that he was taking for his heart. Because no autopsy was done, it was impossible for the plaintiff's attorney to prove that Lasix had contributed to his death. The case was dismissed. But what was most intriguing to me was that this "standard of care" was not "standard."

In the end, my own definition of, or criteria for, standard of care is not the minimal level of acceptable care. Rather, it is how I would want my family or myself to be treated if we were ever afflicted by illness. I completely understand that not every person needs to be evaluated and treated as if being written up as the case of the week in *NEJM*, but I do notice that there are different levels of care that patients receive. When my family or I or any of my patients is sick, I would like the optimal level of care, not just the standard of care.

Chapter Twelve

The Finance of Being in Practice

Supply and Demand

My son Sam, seventeen at the time and about halfway through his introduction to economics course in high school, asked me, "How could you not be generating enough revenue to pay all the DEC's bills? What about the rules of supply and demand?"

Knowing that the incidence of type 2 diabetes is closely correlated with the incidence of obesity — by definition a body mass index (BMI) greater than 30 — and that therefore the term "diabesity" had been coined, he went on, "I know from our conversations and my reports for health class on diabetes that the 'diabesity' epidemic is increasing and there are more people with diabetes now than the National Institutes of Health (NIH) projected years ago. One third of our adults and twenty per cent of our children are obese. The amount of diabetes that has actually occurred, not only nationally but also internationally, is greater than expected and currently makes up seven per cent of our country's population and is responsible for almost twenty per cent of our yearly health care expenditures. To make matters even more critical, the incidence of type 2 diabetes is increasing by over one million people per year and it is projected that one third of the kids born in the year 2000 will develop diabetes in their lifetime. Also, type 1 diabetes is increasing, for unclear reasons, by five per cent per year. The supply of patients is high — at least half of your practice is related to the treatment of diabetes — and the demand for endocrinologists is high, since the supply of practicing endocrinologists is decreasing. Then, what is the problem? I would think you would be doing great financially."

After listening to Sam's analysis, and not showing him the hand once, I said, "Sam, this is one time where the rules of supply and demand just do not work. Unfortunately, the people who control the money, i.e., the insurance companies and the government via Medicare and Medicaid, seem not to value financially what we endocrinologists do, especially compared with other disciplines in medicine, and I certainly get no bonus dollars for being on the *Best Doctors* list. I do not take anything out of people or put anything into them, like surgeons do. I do not read x-rays like a radiologist nor give botox like a plastic surgeon nor do lasik surgery like an ophthalmologist. I do not even take off suspicious skin lesions like a dermatologist. I wish I were paid for giving insulin like a hematologist-oncologist is paid for giving chemotherapeutics, but I am not." I was not finished.

"We could do intraoffice ultrasounds and thyroid aspirates, the only procedures that an endocrinologist may consider doing to generate extra revenue, but frankly, there are so many patients in need of endocrine care that we decided it was the best use of our time to serve our community by seeing more patients, instead of doing procedures that invasive radiologists can do — and have time to do. Therefore, I do not have any procedures that could financially compensate the practice to offset all the financially uncompensated hours I spend each and every day, night, and weekend making sure my patients are optimally treated." I was still not finished.

"The patients I see are complicated even to me, a specialist. They require a lot of time, both in and outside the office, to do the job right. Sure, I can see them faster by taking shortcuts and not addressing all their problems and concerns at each visit but that is not my style of practice. I think people deserve a high level of care and I want to treat them the same way I would want you to be treated if you had diabetes or any other medical condition. There are countless details to identify and treat, seemingly with every patient, and I know details matter. I guess I am not willing to change my practice style because, at this time, I am satisfied with the patient care I am delivering and I believe most of my patients are satisfied as well." I was still not finished.

How Do Doctors Get Paid?

I went on to describe to him that before 1992, when the current Medicare fee schedule was signed into law, doctors were paid by insurance companies and Medicare based upon what each physician considered to be "usual, customary, and reasonable fees" for the services that each provided. But, in the late 1980s, given increasing physicians' fees, the private and public payers wanted a more stable, reliable, "rational" fee schedule (i.e., one that they could control?). Therefore, in 1988 the federal government commissioned a Harvard economist, William Hsaio, Ph.D., to quantify how much work physicians do for each of the tasks they perform, everything from trimming toenails to removing warts to treating out-of-control schizophrenics to doing complicated surgical procedures to managing diabetes. He and his cohorts spent several years interviewing and surveying thousands of doctors in different specialties. In the end, they came up with the Research Based Relative Value Scale (RBRVS), which is a system for describing, quantifying, and reimbursing physician services relative to one another.

The RBRVS is a complex system that takes into account three aspects of physician service: physician work (a function of time spent, judgment, mental effort, technical skill, physical effort, and stress); physician expense; and professional liability insurance. A relative value unit (RVU) is assigned to each of these components for each task. The formula therefore looks like this:

work RVU + practice expense RVU + professional liability
insurance RVU = total RVU

After the total RVU is calculated, it is then multiplied by a conversion factor (CF), which is an actual dollar amount. In 2007 it was $37.8975. The RVU multiplied by the CF is then translated into a current procedural terminology (CPT) code, which is actuallly used to pay doctors for whatever services they have delivered. But that is not all.

A geographical adjustment factor (GAF), known as a

geographic practice cost index (GPCI), is then added into each variable in the total RVU equation. Therefore, the Total RVU equation really looks like this:

[(work RVU x work GPCI) + (practice expense RVU x practice expense GPCI) + (liability RVU x liability GPCI)] x conversion factor = Medicare payment

Are you still with me? Good, because we are still not done. The codes are always changing.

When a new code is approved through the CPT process, it is then sent to the AMA Relative Value Update Committee (called the RUC, not the RVUC) for valuation. If the RUC approves a code, and assigns a dollar amount to that code, then it has to subtract money from another code, because the process must be budget neutral. Therefore, with the budget neutrality work adjuster (BNWA), the new equation looks like this:

[(work RVU x BNWA x work GPCI) + (practice expense RVU x practice expense GPCI) + (liability RVU x liability GPCI)] x conversion factor = Medicare payment

You may be interested to know that there are over 10,000 values for each of the three RVU categories, as well as hundreds of GPCI values, resulting in billions of potential combinations for physicians' fees. According to the Vanderbilt University Medical Center Office of Compliance and Corporate Integrity, there were 645 code changes in 2007, including 258 new codes, 79 revised codes, and 308 codes deleted. Thus the total number of codes in 2007 was 8,611, compared with 8,661 in 2006. We are almost done.

Medicare uses yet another calculation, called the sustainable growth rate (SGR), in an attempt to moderate its spending on physician services. Medicare sets spending targets each year, but if its actual spending on physician services, based on volume and complexity, exceeds predetermined targets for spending that year, then it reduces its payments to physicians.

From 2000 to 2005, Medicare spending for physician services was greater than the targets. Attempts to lower physicians' fees were thwarted by our medical societies' loud protests. In the end the Medicare reimbursement fees stayed essentially flat (increasing by just less than one per cent per year). To spare Sam, I did not go into how hospitals are reimbursed for inpatient care based upon diagnostic related groups (DRGs), which is a whole other story.

Sam now understood that there is no variable within any of these formulas that takes into account physician supply and demand, and that a shortage of endocrinologists and an increasing number of people with diabetes does not mean that we are paid better. Doctors who participate with insurance companies and Medicare are not playing in a free market system like other businesses do. How we get paid is according to what the "other team" decides.

There is also nothing in these formulas that takes disease prevention into account. Rather, in a perverse way, physicians are paid much better for doing more procedures and treating disease than for preventing it. According to the Healthy Lifestyles and Prevention (HeLP) America Act of 2004, "The United States spends over $1,800,000,000,000 annually on health care, 75 percent of which is spent on the treatment of chronic disease. However, only 2 percent of annual health care spending in the United States goes toward the prevention of chronic diseases." But HeLP America, which was designed "to improve the health of Americans and reduce health care costs by reorienting the Nation's health care system towards prevention, wellness, and self care," did not become law. Think how much money could be saved if prevention were made a priority. In the world of diabetes alone, according to the Centers for Disease Control (CDC), about sixty-six diabetics lost their eyesight, 122 people started dialysis, 225 had amputations, and 614 died *each day* due to their diabetes, at a cost of 174 billion dollars in 2007. All these conditions are preventable by either keeping people from developing diabetes or maximizing their treatment if they do develop it. I made less money per hour, trying to prevent diabetes and its complications, than a hospitalist who took care of people once they got sick.

Sam also better understood that we are not paid like

other professionals, such as lawyers and accountants, who are paid by time, whether their clients visit them or not. He also understood that there was nothing in the formula for the time that a physician or nurse may take to talk on the phone with a patient. Nor was there anything in the formula that took into account the time I would take to discuss a case with another doctor or to review correspondence from another doctor about a patient's care. Certainly there was no reimbursement to review lab or test results when the patient was not physically present in the office, or for me to give instructions to the nurse to call the patient with test results. In the past, when reimbursements were better and office expenses were lower, doctors were happy to throw in all this extra stuff for free. But in my case, these throw-ins undermined the sustainability of my practice.

Sam, like most other Americans, was unaware of how physicians are paid; but, like fifty-four per cent of about 1100 patients who responded to the survey reported by Audiey C. Kao, Alan M. Zaslavsky, *et al.*, in the March 2001 *Journal of General Internal Medicine*, he wanted to know. To understand the situation better, he wanted some real numbers and real-life examples.

Real-Life Examples

As an endocrinologist I would spend at least twenty minutes with each diabetic patient, meticulously and tediously going over the details of diabetes management, including how to eat, drink, exercise, take insulin, store insulin, where to inject it, how much to take when well, and how much when sick. I would review with them how to manage their insulin if their blood sugars were too high and how to treat blood sugars if they were too low.

Also, to maximize their care, I wanted to make sure that their blood pressures and cholesterol levels were optimally managed, that they were up to date on their eye exams and kidney tests, and that they had no coronary or peripheral vascular symptoms. Because diabetes can affect general physical and emotional health, and vice versa, I would review these issues with them as well, making sure that they had their vaccinations, colonoscopies, mammograms, and prostate exams. I also made sure that they were taking, tolerating — and affording — all their prescribed medications.

I made myself available to answer any questions that a patient may have had from reading Internet sites or pharmaceutical advertisements. Then it was time for a thorough physical examination. I liked to do a thorough exam at every routine office visit, because exam findings can change between visits. This exam, especially checking the feet, would reassure both the patient and me that everything was OK. I cannot begin to tell you how many patients would say, "Oh, my feet are fine," only for me to discover some big open sore or cut that they had not noticed or could not feel. I would follow the exam with both verbal and written instructions, because studies show that most patients forget much of whatever is told to them at the doctor's office. Thus I preferred to get things in writing for them.

Immediately after I saw a patient, and before I saw the next patient and went through the same routine again — sometimes twenty times a day, regularly five days a week, at least forty-six weeks a year — I would either review the note that my nurse had recorded during the visit or dictate a progress note, which are equally thorough and can be as long as two pages, single-spaced. Such notes document what transpired at each office visit. Although the time and energy to dictate and transcribe these notes was not reimbursable via RVU formulas, I still liked my notes to be thorough, because they enabled me to remember little personal stuff that the patients might have told me, such as vacation trips or happy events in their lives, which I could mention at subsequent visits to let them know that I was listening to them and paying attention to their details.

A thorough note also helped me better to understand each patient's medical care at the next office visit. Last but not least, a thorough note could prove invaluable in a lawsuit or if an insurance company sent in "their team" to verify that my CPT coding was correct and not overcoded, which could result in significant financial penalties. Evidently it is OK if I undercode, because the insurance companies never say, "We owe you money ..."

For all this, I would likely receive between about $75 and $100, far less than a surgical subspecialist might get for doing a simple office procedure, even if both took about the same amount of time.

Sam interrupted me, "But Dad, why are those doctors so much better reimbursed than you? Are they smarter than you? More talented than you? Is what they do more dangerous? Did they spend more time in training than you? Can't people with diabetes get real sick or even die if they are not treated appropriately? I don't understand the disparity in pay."

I responded, "I certainly didn't make up the RVU rules, but if I want to be in a conventional fee-for-service clinical practice I have to play by them. The p(l)aying field is uneven and the teams are unequal. However, I certainly don't begrudge the amount of money that other doctors make. They are playing by the rules also. I don't even resent the $75 or $100 that my practice receives as reimbursement for my services. The problem is that, in order for me to see one patient, it costs the practice, including my salary, more than the $75 or $100 reimbursement. Thus, with each patient, my employer, FPA, actually loses money."

Several years ago, an internist colleague of mine was working for a health maintenance organization (HMO). One day the business manager called him into his office to give him a talking-to about the finances of medicine. He told my friend that he was taking too much time with his patients and that he needed to see patients more quickly. When my friend replied that he needed that much time to give his patients optimal treatments, the business manager rebuffed him and quipped, "You care too much about the patients and if you continue to do so, we'll go broke."

Data from the Martin Fletcher 2007 *Physician Compensation Report* <www.martinfletcher.com> shows that the top six best-paid medical specialists were invasive cardiologists, at number one, earning on average $460,000 per year, then, in order, radiologists, orthopedic surgeons, gastroenterologists, urologists, and, at number six, averaging $337,000 per year, anesthesiologists. Endocrinologists' average salaries are between $175,000 and $199,000, depending on where they practice in the U.S..

Medical Economics Looked at a Little Differently

Sam is not only a huge sports fan, but also enjoys comedians, so I gave him another example of general economics. In March 2005 I went see one of my favorite comedians, Jerry Seinfeld, at the Landmark Theatre in downtown Syracuse. While I sat in this large, beautifully renovated auditorium waiting for the show to start, I looked at my ticket stub, which said $75. Then I looked around and saw that the house was filled to capacity, i.e., about 3000 people; and this was to be Jerry's second show.

I did some quick calculations. If I were to treat three patients per hour in my office, one at a time, eight hours per day, five days per week, forty-six weeks per year, that would be 5520 people, or about 2500 more than were sitting in the Landmark *right now!* Seinfeld would spend about one hour telling his wonderful jokes and stories to everyone at once. In just one night, just two shows, at $75 a head he would bring in more revenue than I would *all year!* Moreover, there would be nobody at the end of the show saying, "Jerry, could you please repeat that one joke? I didn't understand it," or, "Jerry, could you write that down for me since I'm sure I'll forget it by the time I get home?" My advice to Sam was that it is better to "make 'em laugh" than to cry over trying to survive as a clinical endocrinologist.

If You Are a Good Doc You Will Not Have to Be Concerned With Finances

When I finished my endocrine fellowship in 1991, we presumed that, if we did well treating our patients, then everything would work itself out financially. Well, it did not happen quite that way. Most doctors have no formal business training; but to survive complex financial times, they must now master the art of business in addition to the art of medicine. Many of us, in the little spare time we have, are forced to choose between attending continuing medical education (CME) courses for the good of our patients and medical business courses for the good of our businesses. This is while medical research is being published faster than most of us have time to read it. One of my more painful and demoralizing sights was watching the pile of unread medical journals accumulating on my shelf waiting to be read. Sometimes I received between five and ten journals or medical newspapers in just a week. Many times I was too exhausted at the end of the day or during the weekends to read even the titles of the articles. I used to promise myself that on my next vacation I would read through them, but, just like the best intentions of a New Year's resolution, I failed to keep those promises.

To keep up with medical literature some physicians purchase the equivalent of medical crib notes, i.e., we subscribe to newsletters wherein other doctors summarize articles that they have read and that they think are important to us so that we can cut to the chase with new research and get just the bottom line to save us time and still stay current.

We hire expensive business experts and billing specialists to help us try to navigate and survive the system, which adds to our cost of doing business. But who could live without them? What doctor could remember all the billing codes and changes in the rules that seem to take place regularly and still keep up with all the patients that need to be seen and all the medical journals that need to be read each week?

Many new physicians opt to join established groups as employed physicians rather than start their own practices and incur the enormous start-up costs of technologically advanced medicine. This is true for the vast majority of doctors who have accumulated significant debt from undergraduate and medical schools. Even some doctors who had been in solo practice for many years, to the dismay of their patients who loved the personal touch of a mom-and-pop type small practice, have capitulated and joined larger groups. Some doctors simplify by splitting off from larger groups to open small boutique practices that each serve only a fortunate few who can afford to pay out of pocket for their care. Thus doctors can limit their practices to a few hundred patients each instead of a few thousand. But among the risks of boutique practices is not only that they further restrict access to primary care physicians, but also that they may create a two-tiered medical system, one for the wealthy, the other for the not-so-wealthy and the poor.

Some doctors from different disciplines join together to form large multi-specialty groups to try to maximize their economies of scale, reduce their expenses, and be in better positions to bargain reimbursements with the insurance companies. Docs from separate practices cannot discuss the prices they respectively charge, given the antitrust laws — yet somehow these laws do not seem to apply to insurance companies.

Two of my experienced staff were hired away from my practice because we could not give them their deserved raises. They were bought out by what I refer to as the "New York Yankees doctors," in this case hematology-oncology and pain management physicians, who performed procedures and therefore generated greater revenues than I did. They could afford to pay nurses better than we could, the "Kansas City Royals doctors," non-procedural, lower revenue generating physicians. This was after we had spent years training these nurses, getting them up to the major league level. We then had to go back to the minor leagues of nursing, to find less experienced, less expensive nurses, and then go through the entire training process again.

To assist their incomes, some doctors buy or erect office buildings and buy or lease MRI scanners, x-ray machines, lab instruments, and other testing devices. Most cannot generate enough revenue to cover expenses from just seeing patients. Each year physicians' expenses increase, including malpractice premiums, health care costs, EMR, and staff salaries. The DEC's expenses just to keep a part-time nurse practitioner,

a part-time endocrinologist, and myself in practice for one year
was over a million dollars. That is a lot of $75 office visits. In
football vernacular we called this "grinding it out," trying to
gain one or two yards with each patient visit. But we had no
big plays to score a financial touchdown.

We at FPA had a lab. If we had not, I doubt that our
practice could have afforded to stay open for a month. The lab
not only helped to generate revenue, but also added to patient
convenience. Unfortunately we had to negotiate — i.e., fight
— with many different insurance companies to get approval
for our patients to come to our own lab, because the insurance
companies had already made financial arrangements with other
labs to do the work at lower prices, so that the insurance companies could make greater profits. These outside labs took
lower payment for each test in exchange for being guaranteed
a greater volume of tests.

Why else but for money would insurance companies
negotiate lower rates wherever they could? They certainly did
not care about the convenience of the patients. It was not at all
convenient for patients to have to leave my office, where they
could have had their labs done and been out the door in ten
minutes. Instead, they had to pack up all their stuff and drive
some distance, taking up more of their time, just so the insurance companies could make more money. That hardly seemed
fair. Were the patients just pawns in the insurance game? I
thought they were living people, human beings with feelings
and emotions. Doctors are supposed to help them, not just
profit from them, or allow others to profit from them.

If patients had to go to an outside lab, I was still responsible for interpreting their test results, calling them or
having my nurses call them with the test results, and making
changes in their medical management as necessary. Yet, our
reimbursement for that was *zero*! I suppose that I could have
had the patients come in to review the lab tests to generate
more revenue, like some of my endocrine colleagues did, but
I just could not justify inconveniencing the patients again, by
having them leave their jobs or homes, maybe getting babysit-
ters, driving all the way to the office, sitting in the waiting room,

possibly as long as thirty minutes, just so I could tell them that their labs looked fine or make simple changes in their medications. Why bring them in for anything that could easily be accomplished with simple phone calls? Call me a fool, but I tried to respect their time and, if I could make their days easier, then I would do it.

I did not care much about doing the work for nothing, because my motto always was "Patients matter most." However, at least in part, my practice closed because of all the financially uncompensated time. That was a shame, given the abundance of endocrine-related diseases and the shortage of endocrinologists.

Do You Really Want to Be an Endocrinologist?

"Endocrinology Shortage Worsens" was the title of Jane Anderson's lead story in the February 2007 issue of *Clinical Endocrinology News*. She cited several articles, studies, and interviews that described the crisis as it has unfolded since 1995 and as projected to 2020. Demand for endocrinologists is increasing as the nation becomes fatter, flabbier, and unhealthier, but supply is dwindling, in part because of systematic, political, and economic pressures on new doctors *not* to specialize in endocrinology. Positive incentives to enter this field are simply not there. Endocrinology residency positions remain about eleven per cent unfilled each year. The absolute number of new endocrinologists fell each year from 1995 to 1999. Nonmedical hassles of clinical practice, especially from insurance companies, prompt significant numbers of endocrinologists to retire early. One endocrinology leader interviewed for Anderson's article estimated that in 2007 the shortage was fifteen per cent, while another suggested that, even if there were twice as many endocrinologists in our country, they would all have plenty to do. Anderson and her interviewees concluded that, although endocrinology is a fascinating field, it continues underpopulated, and its patients underserved, mainly because of unfair reimbursements.

The ADA Web site <www.diabetes.org> reported on September 13, 2006, that the Hospital Association of Pennsylvania in 2005 showed a statewide twenty-two per cent endocrinologist vacancy rate and that the American Association of Clinical Endocrinologists (AACE) showed a nationwide rate of twelve per cent — the highest vacancy rate for any medical specialty.

To be trained in internal medicine and specialize in endocrinology, we have to complete four years of undergraduate work, four years of medical school, one year of internship, then two years of residency followed by a fellowship, which could be as many as two or three additional years of training. Along the way, we have to pass numerous certification exams. Some of these tests take as long as two days to complete and cost upward of $1000, not including the travel, hotel, and food.

After these thirteen or fourteen years of training and incurring significant debt to pay for all this education, we then have the privilege of working long hours and dealing with some of the most complicated and challenging medical conditions. Then, every ten years, we have to recertify to remain credentialed to practice endocrinology. Our senior doctors are grandfathered. They do not have to retake these difficult, time-consuming, and expensive tests; although one might think that if anyone should recertify, it should be those who have been out of training the longest. Note that although doctors, lawyers, and certified public accountants have to take continuing education classes each year, lawyers and CPAs do not have to retake the bar exam or the CPA exam every ten years.

Trying to Sell Endocrinology to the Next Generation

In 2007 I was invited to talk at our local medical school on the virtues of being an endocrinologist. The meeting was open to all first and second-year medical students, about 300 students. About ten or twelve students showed up. I told them many of the reasons why I went into endocrinology, including loving what I do, the incredibly interesting and different cases, the great professors, and my own predilection to enjoy taking on very difficult challenges. In that regard, I was totally satisfied with my choice to be an endocrinologist. However, when the topic of reimbursement and time commitment came up, I gave these students my honest opinion. Several of them left the meeting before it was scheduled to end. My experience was not unique, as Miriam E. Tucker's article, "Most U.S. Medical Students Reject Careers in Diabetes Care," plainly showed in *Clinical Endocrinology News*, September 2008.

Do You Really Want to Be a Primary Care Provider?

There was an advertisement in a 2007 issue of *NEJM* from a hospital looking for five different specialists. It gave the starting salaries as follows: family practitioner $140,000, internist $150,000, rheumatologist $190,000, pulmonologist $220,000, and radiologist $350,000. Why does the radiologist start with two and a half times the salary of the internist?

I acknowledge that these are all excellent salaries, especially compared with the average American worker, but my father used to say, "Nobody pays you that kind of money for nothing." We physicians worked extremely hard to become physicians, with significant financial outlay, years of incredibly intense education and training, endless testing, and enormous personal sacrifices. There are so many other ways that people can make a buck that require much less time, expense, or personal sacrifice than going through a medical training program, not to mention the continued threat of malpractice every time we see a patient. Just ask the bankers and brokers on Wall Street how easy it was to make big bucks before the implosion of our financial system in late 2008.

In my day and before, the top of the class went into the practice of general internal medicine. At that time the surgical residents called us medical residents "fleas," because we were all over our patients, knowing all the excruciating details about their medical conditions. But now, we internists might be called "fleas" for a different reason. We are undervalued among medical specialists, as evidenced by disparate pay and lifestyles. Now our best and brightest are dissuaded from entering cognitive medical fields like internal medicine, family practice, psychiatry, general pediatrics, pediatric rheumatology, neuro-ophthalmology, and endocrinology. One just does not get paid as well for thinking.

There was only one graduating senior resident from the 2009 internal medicine program at Upstate Medical University who pursued a career in general internal medicine. When I queried many of the other medical residents who were pursuing specialty careers about why they were not going into general internal medicine, they almost uniformly responded that it was disrespected and financially undervalued. They added that generalists do the work that nobody else wants to do, like filling out disability and insurance forms, and that to know fully all the nuances that are necessary to practice excellent general internal medicine is quite difficult, unlike some other medical specialties and subspecialties, where the information needed for excellence is more limited.

I do not blame medical students for pursuing higher-paying fields of medicine, especially if they enjoy those disciplines. The son of one of my best friends, an orthopedic surgeon, chose orthopedics because he saw all the good that his father did and would like to be in practice with him some day. But some may be pushed into lucrative fields just to pay off the significant debts that they accrued during their training. Others may just be attracted to the relatively enormous amounts of money that can be made. What disquiets me is the significant disparity among what various kinds of physicians earn. Why should that be? We all take significant risks in treating our patients.

In 2008 I reviewed a case for a malpractice defense attorney. An internist had prescribed a commonly used antibiotic, levofloxacin, for a seemingly innocent upper respiratory infection in a woman who had myasthenia gravis. Hidden deep, very deep, in the *Physicians' Desk Reference* (PDR), in the finest of print, were instructions not to give this antibiotic to patients with myasthenia gravis unless there were no alternatives, because doing so may cause respiratory arrest with potential for sudden death. That is exactly what happened to this patient. Being a doctor is a dangerous game no matter what your specialty is.

I know some internists and family practitioners who have taken part-time jobs in addition to their full-time practices, such as working in nursing homes or hospitals all night and then working in their offices all the next day. Why? To supplement their declining incomes caused by declining reimbursements. Is this the reward that doctors should reap for the sacrifices that they made to survive the intense competition to get the highest grades in undergraduate and medical school, internship, and residency: having to work two jobs? Alternatively, maybe they should read *Your Money or Your Life*.

In "Piecework: Medicine's Money Problem," a major article in the *New Yorker* of April 4, 2005, Atul Gawande cited Dartmouth professor William Weeks's findings that, in general, physicians work longer hours than other professionals, averaging close to sixty hours per week, and their return on investment, from the cost of going to college and professional school, was lower for a family practitioner (sixteen per cent) than for a general surgeon (eighteen per cent), a lawyer (twenty-three per cent), or a businessperson with an M.B.A. (twenty-six per cent). Gawande added that "a 2004 survey of Massachusetts physicians found that fifty-eight per cent were dissatisfied with the trade-off between their income and the number of hours they were working; fifty-six per cent thought their income was not competitive with what others earn in comparable professions; and forty per cent expected to see their income fall over the next five years."

I admit that I earned a good income when I was in practice, even though I did not have a raise for four years, and I am not complaining. However, it is not hard to guess why a medical student, especially one burdened with significant debt, would choose a field like radiology over primary care or endocrinology. It is also not hard to understand why there is, and will continue to be, an increasing shortage of primary care doctors and endocrinologists in our nation unless this pay disparity changes.

Dermatology Sounds Better, No?

Natasha Singer's feature in the March 19, 2008, *New York Times* on the yearly ritual of Match Day, whereby medical students are assigned to residency programs, told of a husband and wife team, at the top of their Harvard Medical School class, who were each lucky enough to be accepted into a dermatology program. Singer wrote: "Only 61 percent of seniors at American medical schools whose first choice was dermatology received a residency in that field last year, compared with 98 percent for those whose first choice was internal medicine and 99 percent for those seeking family medicine." Another telling sentence in her article was "'It is an unfortunate circumstance that you can spend an hour with a patient treating them for diabetes and hypertension and make $100, or you can do Botox and make $2,000 in the same time', said Dr. Eric C. Parlette, 35, a dermatologist in Chestnut Hill, Mass."

E. Ray Dorsey *et al.* reported in the September 3, 2003, *JAMA* that the average dermatologist worked 45.5 hours per week, compared with 52.5 hours for a family practitioner and 57.0 for an internist. Yet the 2004 AMGA Medical Group Compensation and Financial Survey showed a decline of 1.81 per cent in internists' compensation, compared with increases of 16.71 per cent for dermatologists and 7.05 per cent for family practitioners. The 2006 data from the same survey had the income of internists and family practitioners each up just over eight per cent, and that of dermatologists up about twelve per cent, still leading the pack.

In "Physician Career Satisfaction Across Specialties" by J. Paul Leigh *et al.* in the July 22, 2002, *Archives of Internal Medicine*, dermatology ranked as the third most satisfying medical specialty. Internal medicine ranked last — but *geriatric* internal medicine ranked first.

The Easterlin paradox asserts that what is important

to people is not their *absolute* income, but their *relative* income, compared with that of others. This may be most obvious with our elite professional athletes. They each want more money than their peers, because the highest paid is judged the best. But it is true in medicine too. I admit that I felt some distress each day when I arrived at the office before and left after the dermatologist down the hall. I knew that those skin docs were making much more than I was. I feel guilty to admit this, because my family and I were OK financially, but, as my mom used to say, "Feelings are feelings, they are neither right nor wrong. They just are." It seems that Easterlin at least had me pegged right. How would you feel?

Physician Competing Against Physician

Physicians' incomes accounted for only twenty-two per cent of the 2.1 trillion dollars spent on health care in the U.S. in 2006, as Maggie Mahar reported at <www.healthbeatblog. org/2008/01/health-care-s-1.html>.

Very distressing to me and my colleagues is that the insurance companies, by decreasing reimbursements and increasing patient premiums, have commandeered more money than ever. Sometimes people ask me why I became a physician and I answer — half kidding — that it was cheaper to become a doctor and treat myself than to pay all the co-pays, deductibles, and premiums that insurance companies require when a patient sees a physician. Where does all the premium and co-pay money go? I guarantee that it is not coming to physicians in the form of higher reimbursements.

In 2006, fees to physicians from private insurers, on average, were lower than government-run, not-for-profit Medicare, according to Moore in her January 2007 article in *Physicians Practice*. Because, as I described earlier in this chapter, Medicare fees have been rather flat since 2000, one can only deduce that private insurances have been paying physicians less. Moore also reports that United, WellPoint, and Aetna, the top three insurers, control seventy-three per cent of the

106 million people insured by the top ten health insurers, i.e., 77.7 million, thus giving them significant leverage over us, the physicians. It also distresses me to see large advertisements from the insurance companies on billboards, in newspapers, and on the TV. This marketing money could be so much better spent on actually delivering health care.

Given the flat or lower fee schedules, physicians also compete against each other for the same piece of the money pie. We are supposed to be on the same team. Physician competes against physician, sorry to say, trying to squeeze every dollar they can from their respective patients to make up for their declining revenues, so that they do not end up like the DEC. For example, tests that used to be done by cardiologists and neurologists, like echocardiograms and nerve conduction velocities, are now done in primary care offices.

In my office we did a non-invasive procedure called an ankle-brachial index (ABI) to try to determine if a person, who complained of pains in the legs while walking, had diminished blood flow to the legs. The nurses did the study and calculated the results. I gave additional instructions to the patient, based on these results, which took just seconds to obtain. The charge was $261, a fortune compared to the $75 or $100 that I received for twenty minutes face-to-face evaluating a person with diabetes. One might ask, "Why not do ABIs on everyone?" The answer was that not everyone needed the test. Yet it would have been a relatively easy way to prop up the bottom line.

I totally believe in the free market and free enterprise. Competition and capitalism create more skillful people and better products. However, the attraction for the dollar is so strong that it can be distorting to all, including physicians. Even hospitals are caught up in the competition. In our small city, Syracuse, one hospital touts itself as "Medicine at its Best." Another responds with "Simply the Best." Another's slogan is "The Heart Hospital." Even our VA hospital is involved. Its slogans are "Leading Health Care into the Twenty-First Century" and "The Price of Freedom Can Be Seen Here."

Remind me again, did we go into medicine to save lives

or to make a killing? Remember, the commodity I am talking about is people and their health. I hope we are not using them as pawns. To have all their tests done in one location is a definite convenience for patients; but I am mystified as to whether physicians do tests in their offices for patient convenience, for necessity in good patient care, for defensive medicine to reduce the liability risk, for the income, or for all or some of the above.

Resneck, Lipton, and Pletcher stated in the December 2007 issue of the *Journal of the American Academy of Dermatology* that, if patients want botox injections, then their wait time to see a dermatologist is about one week. But, if they have suspicious skin lesions that need evaluation, then their wait time would be three or four weeks. What conclusions would you draw from the results of this study? My daughter was home from college one summer for only a short period of time. We tried to get an appointment with her dermatologist to treat her acne. No way. We should have said that she needed some cosmetic surgery. We might have then heard, "Bring her in this afternoon." Note that patients who order elective cosmetic procedures tend to pay cash at time of service, but patients who actually need to see a doctor tend to rely on insurance, thus creating more paperwork and headaches for the doctor's staff.

A few of our local gynecologists purchased a certain bone densitometer to evaluate women for osteoporosis and did bone density studies on this machine, even though some of their patients had had bone density studies done in the past on other brands of densitometers. It is almost impossible to compare studies done on two different companies' densitometers. Thus, these physicians could not tell these patients with any certainty whether the inconvenient and cumbersome osteoporosis treatments that they were taking were helping. Insurance companies would pay for a bone density study only every two years. So, unless each patient were willing to pay about $150 out of pocket to repeat the test on the previous densitometer, they would each have to wait an additional two years before learning the efficacy of their treatments.

Radiologists also do bone density studies on their own

machines, without asking if patients had any previous bone density studies done on different densitometers, thus putting patients in the same situation as with those gynecologists. I would routinely try to send patients back to the same radiologists for follow-up bone density studies, so as to try to have each study done on the same densitometer (or at least the same brand of densitometer) to improve the accuracy of test comparisons. Sometimes, however, between the last and the current study, the radiologist would have bought a different densitometer, and would do the follow-up on the new one, even though any eighth-grade general science student could tell you that comparing successive data from two different machines is mostly useless. Thus the patients were left not knowing whether their osteoporosis treatments were working or not.

Are these gynecologists and radiologists greedy, ignorant, or just apathetic about this situation?

In 2006 Medicare unilaterally proposed reducing the reimbursement for any future bone density study to only about $40, which soured the investments of those physicians who had already purchased densitometers to try to supplement their incomes. This is another example of why I was skittish to open my own office and practice solo, even though I considered it many times, thinking that it might be good for my patients. We physicians can never plan financially for the future when the rules arbitrarily and suddenly change without any input from us. The insurance companies or Medicare never seem to say, "Hey, docs, what would you think if we cut your reimbursements? Would that be OK with you? Would you mind discussing it with us? ..."

Marketing Sells, Even for Doctors

Because of the system of declining reimbursements, doctors now are advertising on radio, billboards, TV, and the Internet to get patients for cosmetic surgeries, eye refraction procedures like lasik, hair restoration, etc. Such an ad could go something like this:

For me, an idealist, who went into medicine for pure (naïve?) reasons, it is sad to see our ancient and noble profession moving in this direction. Patients used to go to doctors because of reputation and skill, not because of catchier advertising.

Pay for Performance

I suspect that we try to squeeze more from our patients as the insurance companies try to squeeze more from us. There is a concept called "pay for performance." The idea is that, if we do a better job taking care of our diabetics, for example, then the insurance companies pay us more. Or rather, is it that they pay us the same and penalize the doctors who do not perform as well? The marker for successful treatment of people with diabetes is a blood test called hemoglobin A1c, which measures the average glucose over each previous three months. On first look, this seemed like a good idea — as I certainly enjoy some good competition along with better medical care for our patients.

The problem is that the idea was flawed in at least three fundamental ways.

First, the hemoglobin A1c test is not 100 per cent accurate. Frankly, no test is. Several conditions could falsely raise or lower the result — and what if the patients do not even come in for their quarterly checkups?

Second, what would doctors do if their patients were not able to improve their hemoglobin A1c tests because they could not afford the medications — which is not inconceivable, given the high cost of medications in the U.S., compared with other countries? What if the medications had side effects that the patients could not tolerate? What if the patients just were not willing to do the things necessary to improve their blood sugars, like diet and exercise? Two thirds of people with diabetes have hemoglobin A1c levels higher than the ADA goals. Would good docs ask such patients to leave their practices just because they would drain their finances? Where would they go? Who would want them if they were financial disincentives? Would docs try to replace them with "good diabetics" who would be more compliant?

Third, although many patients and insurance companies want transparent disclosure of physician outcomes, the ability to collect this data accurately and reliably comes into question. For example, insurance companies in my area would phone my patients to ask them when they had their last hemoglobin A1c, eye, cholesterol, or microalbumin checks. With all due respect, many patients are unable to recall these details or, despite education and discussion, do not really know what these tests are. Frankly, I too have difficulty remembering when I had my last physical exam or dental cleaning. Other times, insurance company personnel would come into my office to review charts, looking for information, but either not finding it or flat-out missing it. Such pitfalls surely affect whatever data is obtained. A popular and well-reputed physician incentive program is offered by Bridges to Excellence (BTE) <www. bridgestoexcellence.org>, "a not-for-profit organization created to encourage significant leaps in the quality of care by recognizing and rewarding health care providers who demonstrate that they deliver safe, timely, effective, efficient, equitable and patient-centered care." As of June 2009 it was available in only twenty-two states, but as its message gains strength so does its popularity. What seems ironic to me is that physicians are given such financial incentives to do what we should be doing anyway. In the end, however, the coach's or the doctor's wins and losses can only be as good as their players' or patients' desires and abilities to carry out the plays or to follow instructions. Victory for all comes when the team works as a single unit.

No Health Insurance = Roulette

As of March 2008, NIH data showed that we had over forty-seven million people in this country without health insurance. The number was just under forty million in 1993. Moreover, the number of uninsured rises about a million for every one per cent that the unemployment rate rises. As this book comes to press in June 2009, the national unemployment rate is pushing nine per cent, the worst since 1983, and a rise of over four per cent in less than two years. A one in three chance exists that even people with health insurance will be without it at some time over the next three years. Seeing any uninsured patient in my office raised the degree of difficulty of treating that patient to another level. It was time-consuming to find out the costs of their medications, because the same medicines had different costs at different pharmacies. It was even harder to find out the actual costs of labs or tests ordered, because different laboratories had different charges for the same tests, and these figures were not easily obtainable.

I was even more careful of the tests that I ordered for

uninsured patients, asking myself, "Do I really, really, really need that information to help this patient?" I would try to balance this with the possibility of missing a diagnosis and having full liability. Not only would I feel terrible if something bad were to happen to a patient, but also, I could not imagine a judge or jury saying to me after one of my uninsured patients had had a bad outcome, "Don't worry about it, Doc. He had no money anyway. You are free to go."

Also not clear was what the actual charges would be if a patient went to an ER or was admitted to the hospital. No prices are listed in hospitals as they are in take-out restaurants. The patient does not say, "Hmmmm, I'll take an IV with saline, an EKG with some lab work, but hold the chest x-ray, I just can't afford it today."

Patients without insurance may be expected to pay the actual "usual, customary, and reasonable fees" that physicians or hospitals charge, which is much more than the watered-down amounts that insurance companies typically pay the providers. Doctors' charges to insurance companies are normally inflated, because, if we charged insurance companies less than what they were willing to pay, then they would just pay us even less than that.

In April 2006, New York State passed a law, effective January 1, 2007, to try to protect the uninsured and underinsured from being overcharged by hospitals. Nevertheless, according to *Hospital Financial Assistance Programs: Are New York Hospitals Complying with New Requirements?*, the March 2008 report of the Public Policy and Education Fund of New York, compliance with this law was poor in its first two years.

Two of my uninsured patients died because they thought that their acute problems would just go away. Mrs. G., an extremely pleasant, rotund woman with short gray hair and a winning smile, had diabetes, hypertension, hypothyroidism, and vascular disease. She called our office one Wednesday afternoon to say that she had a cold, with fevers and a productive cough. We offered her an office visit for that afternoon, but, given her financial situation and her lack of insurance, she just wanted us to call in an antibiotic (which, of course, would not work on a viral cold). "It's just a virus," she insisted, "I'll be OK."

We phoned her the next day to check on her, because she lived alone and had limited social supports. She sounded worse. We once again offered her an office visit for that day, and even begged her to either come in or go to the ER. She once again refused and reassured me that she would be OK. We called her again on Friday and the same scene played out. The next time I heard about her was when her picture showed up in the obituaries that Sunday morning. Her lack of health insurance cost her life.

My other patient who died from not having health insurance was transgender, male-to-female. I had known Ms. K. for years. When we first met she was living as a male, married with two children, and working as an executive in a major company. She had excellent health insurance and, overall, a stable financial situation. She was referred to my practice by her therapist. We all agreed that the time was finally right for her to make the gender switch, something she had been contemplating since childhood.

It was liberating for her to start becoming who she always wanted to be, although, as you may imagine, there were many significant social hurdles, as well as consequences of her decision for her spouse, children, and employment. In the end, her family rejected her and she lost her executive job.

While working odd jobs, all without any insurance coverage, she began having peculiar symptoms, which I thought could be cardiac in origin. I urged her, even pleaded with her several times over several days, to come to the office or go to the ER. She refused. The next I heard about her was a few days after this last conversation, when the medical examiner's office called to say that Ms. K. had been found dead in her apartment.

Rightly or wrongly, I blamed the health insurance CEOs and executives after these two people lost their lives for no reason other than money. I thought about the steady increase in the cost of insurance premiums, at least since 1999, that have rendered it unaffordable for so many. I also thought of the millions of dollars that these executives have taken in salary, stock options, and bonuses — for what? Denying my patients' care and keeping the money for themselves? I recognize that they have not denied them care, just payment, but for Americans without insurance, that amounts to the same thing if they cannot otherwise afford care.

These patients are forced to play roulette with their lives. They are left with the enormous burden of having to decide for themselves, on their own, whether they are sick enough to see a doctor or go to an ER or an urgent care center and spend all that money or, on the other horn of the dilemma, whether they can feel safe waiting it out and hoping that whatever they have will just go away.

Two More of the Forty-Seven Million

Two more cases of people without health insurance are worth mentioning.

On April 12, 2008, a Syracuse family was driving to Florida on I-95 to visit Disney World. Somewhere in South Carolina a drunk driver crashed his vehicle head-on into their minivan. The collision killed fourteen-year-old Samantha Reynolds and left her stepmother, Brenda, critically injured. Once stabilized, Brenda was flown by air ambulance back to Syracuse to be treated. The problem? No health insurance. Imagine going on a long-anticipated family vacation only to have your euphoria destroyed by your stepdaughter's death, your own critical injuries, and having no health insurance.

The community banded together to try to help defray her medical expenses by organizing a can and bottle drive, a raffle, and other fundraising events. *A can and bottle drive?!* How many five-cent cans and bottles do you think it would take to pay for the amount of time in the ICU, the surgical procedures, or the medications and rehab she would need if she survives? Can you count that high?

The second case concerned a healthy young woman who graduated college in 2007. As her "reward," she was no longer able to be covered by her parents' health insurance. As she was physically well but had no money, she took what she considered a small risk that she would not get sick or injured until she had secured a job and obtained health insurance from her new employer.

She did find a job with health insurance as a benefit. But, just weeks before she was to start her new job, her kidneys failed, requiring a kidney transplant. Impeccable timing! She and her family had to hold fundraisers to pay for not only the acute care of the transplant and the associated hospitalization, but also all the follow-up care, including very expensive anti-rejection medications. I am sure now, when she tries to obtain health insurance in the future, she will not be the first round draft pick of any insurance company.

Doctors Make Too Much Money

How much was it worth to someone who suffered cardiac arrest while in the hospital and was shocked back to life? During my residency this scene played out several times. How much was it worth to a pregnant woman with diabetes to have me talk with her on the phone three or four times a week to make sure her blood sugars were optimal and her pregnancy and delivery went along uneventfully? How much was it worth to an insomniac, shaky, jittery person with symptomatic hyperthyroidism and heart palpitations, unable to work, to be treated and to feel normal again? The answers to these questions are all the same: I have no idea, but I was happy to help.

My ophthalmology friend was a panelist during a health care symposium in 2008 and was asked to comment on the return on investment that doctors receive once they finish their medical training. His answer, in part, was that an eye doctor used to need to do about six cataracts to buy a Cadillac, euphemistically called the "cataract to Cadillac ratio." But in 2008 he would have had to do sixty or seventy cataract procedures to buy that Cadillac, which indicated that reimbursement for physicians was going down, compared with the cost of living, or at least compared with the increasing price of Cadillacs.

I believe that we physicians deserve an appropriate income for the time it took us to become doctors and the responsibility and stress associated with the job. However, it seemed always peculiar to me that a patient would pay me money for helping with a most cherished possession: health. Many patients would come in with significant physical or emotional problems, sometimes crying their heads off. Some cried because they hated their jobs but could not leave, because they would lose their health insurance. They could not get new policies, because of "pre-existing conditions"! I was often able to help them with medications, appropriate referrals, or by just being an interested, compassionate listener. Then, at the end of each visit, I would bill them.

It was as if a police officer were to come to my house in the middle of the night because I heard sounds outside, hand me a bill, and say, "Dr. Lebowitz, everything is fine. That's a 'level three' visit. Please remit $50 to the cashier who is conveniently located in the back seat of the patrol car." Or as if the firefighters who saved the lives of your family were to tell you, "That was a very complicated case. That's a 'level five' visit. Please pay the cashier seated in the hook and ladder"? The "business" of medicine should likewise be an oxymoron, like the "business" of police work or firefighting, but it is not.

Some have said that physicians in America make too much money, especially compared with physicians in other countries. Doctors are not supposed to be in it for the money. Yet Gawande in his April 4, 2005, *New Yorker* article cited multiple surveys that showed two thirds of Americans believing that doctors care too much about money. To try to avoid that stereotype, I intentionally kept my cars as long as possible, i.e., until, due to excessive salt used on the snowy and icy roads of Central New York, there was more rust than paint and no one in my family would ride with me. I worried that, if I drove a nicer car, my patients might think that I cared more about money than their health, or that I was charging them too much. But if businesspeople drive nice cars, we think them really successful. I dressed neatly but plainly for the office: buttoned shirt, tie, slacks — and no jewelry except a counterfeit Piaget watch that my father-in-law had given me years ago. I kidded my patients that he gave the real Piaget to his other son-in-law, whom he liked better. I believe that my patients would look at my clothes and feel like I was one of them, not an elitist, and thus could better relate to their troubles.

We were trained to be selfless, if not self-satisfied, during our residency, while we toiled endless hours and were proud to say we made minimum wage. It made us feel like we were doing something difficult and special, genuinely serving humankind without any financial incentives. It was pure. However, once in practice, working extremely long hours with significant stresses, needing to start paying back exorbitant student loans, and seeing how much money insurance company executives were making off our toil and sweat of doing the actual work of patient care, we physicians naturally began to want appropriate incomes.

My Wife is Kicking Me under the Table

Maybe I have said too much. I can imagine, if I were sitting at a table discussing these issues with some friends, that my wife would be kicking me under the table to make me stop talking. I just hate the idea that the insurance companies financially squeeze us physicians, our patients, and business owners with increasing premiums, larger co-pays, and higher deductibles, while making some services more difficult to get — all while they are making so much. We doctors, in turn, squeeze each other and sometimes our patients, so that we too can make a lot and still feel like all the aggravation is worthwhile. Sometimes I feel like we see dollar signs walking into our offices and not people who have diabetes, vascular disease, or depression. I am dismayed that we seem to be acting more and more like businesspeople and less and less like physicians. Where does that leave the patients? Are they just pawns in the game, pieces of plastic on a chess board, whom insurance companies and sometimes even doctors move around so that they can profit from them? Have we taken our eye off the ball as to what is most important? Have we gotten so far off course that money matters more than the people whom we are supposed to be treating?

I will stop now. My wife just kicked me again.

Chapter Thirteen

The Insurance Companies

If It Makes No Sense, They Thought of It (or, If It Makes "Cents," They Thought of It)

Several years ago our high school football team was being clobbered by our opponents — and the referees. In the fourth quarter, with our team well behind and a lopsided defeat imminent, another egregious, unfair penalty was called against our team. One of our usually mild-mannered coaches responded uncharacteristically. He lost it. He snapped. He began yelling and screaming at the top of his lungs in total frustration and despair. "I can't hold it in anymore," he hollered, and went on from there with comments best left for the football field or the locker room. I understand his pain and suffering. I have been enduring similar aggravations and frustrations with the insurance industry since I started practice in 1991 and "I can't hold it in anymore" either.

The insurance companies seem intentionally to have put up so many fences to jump over, oceans to swim, and quicksand to run through, that each day I felt like I was running a steeplechase. It wore me and my staff down — their intention, I am sure. They raised the degree of difficulty to treat my patients to unimaginable levels. They succeeded in making my hard days even harder: "You need preauthorization for this. Send in an appeal for that. Here's an outright rejection for the other." I felt like Oliver Twist when asking "them" for approval for a medication or a test: "Please sir, may I have another?" Then, every time we thought that we understood the rules of their game, they changed them, apparently to maintain their power over us.

I hate to think negatively about anyone. Nevertheless, the insurance industry has left me no choice but to think of them as the opponents, the "other team," the enemy.

What was most infuriating was that many of their rules seemed arbitrary, if not capricious or downright antagonistic.

Their obstacles to patient care seemed intentional, such as long waits on the phone; saying that they had not received a form that we had filled out, even though we had documentation that we had sent it; or just outrightly refusing a test, hoping we would not appeal. Gawande, again in the April 4, 2005, *New Yorker*, said that health insurers would routinely figure out how to deny almost thirty per cent of claims. Perhaps this strategy was just to wear docs and their staffs out so that we would stop trying to order tests or treatments. Then they could simply keep the money that they collected from our patients in the form of premiums.

The more care they deny, the more money they keep. The more care they allow us to provide, the less money they make.

It is appalling that their medical directors have a minimum denial rate that they are supposed to achieve each year and they get bonuses if they exceed that rate. They make more money if they *deny* care to our patients! What is most upsetting is the obvious, profound conflict of interest: To us doctors, patients matter most. To them it appears that money matters most.

I have a saying that I believe characterizes their decision-making, "If it makes no sense medically, they thought of it; if it makes 'cents' financially, they thought of it." I would love to have a one-way mirror to look in on their meetings. While we are busy seeing patients, they probably spend all day conniving and scheming their next steps, thinking that they can do anything they want to us doctors. They probably congratulate themselves with their diabolical Vincent Price laughs, "They're altruistic, we're not! We have the money, they don't! We can collude, they can't! WHAHAHAHA!"

You want examples? I'll give you some from my practice alone. Chew on these inequities and tell me how they taste. I choked on them all day every day for years.

Point Counterpoint

POINT: The insurance company refused to pay for diabetes education and dietary consultation in a patient with very poorly controlled diabetes and significantly increased risk of all the major complications.

COUNTERPOINT: I know that they understand the importance of education for people with diabetes. Everyone knows that this is the centerpiece of all diabetes treatments. However, I suspect the insurance companies of calculating that such patients will likely not develop complications for years and by then may be insured by another insurance company, thus making it someone else's financial problem. We, the physicians, look out for the long-term health of our patients, while each insurance company seems to look out for the short-term financial health of itself.

Also, many insurance companies will not pay for weight loss medications, even though weight loss can significantly improve the blood sugars in patients with type 2 diabetes. As another poke in the doctor's eye, insurance companies hire independent companies to help manage our diabetics outside our offices, sometimes without our approval. Rather than spend that money to hire outside agencies, nurses, or pharmacists, why could they not just reimburse us better, thus enabling us to spend more time with our patients and give them better care? Again, if it makes no sense, they thought of it.

POINT: A patient with type 1 diabetes, who had been on insulin for over twenty years, now all of a sudden needed a letter of necessity from me, stating that she had to be on insulin, in order for her to be reimbursed.

COUNTERPOINT: This was a pure, unadulterated, blatant intrusion. They wanted me to spend time, which I did not have, dictating a letter, and to spend extra money, which the practice did not have, to pay the transcriptionist to send them this letter, indicating that my insulin-dependent diabetic of twenty years needed insulin? How could they justify that request?

By the way, when an insurance company sent a letter to me for additional information, it was not signed by a person. Rather, it was from the pharmacy or the medical records department. No names were given, so, if we wanted a specific person to contact, we could not have one. They know everything about us, our education, certifications, and prescribing habits, but we know nothing about them, not even the identity of the writers of the letters they send. Are they hiding? They behave like the Wizard of Oz, arrogant, hubristic, believing themselves to be all-powerful, but still hiding behind a curtain. Are they too embarrassed to be known? Does their behavior show lack of shame and loss of integrity?

POINT: The insurance company denies coverage for certain diagnoses. But when you call, speak with their personnel, and ask for a specific diagnosis code, they obscure the patient's problem and say, "Oh, we can't tell you that." In other instances they approve the test but do not guarantee payment; i.e., they may decide later, after the test is done, that they do not want to pay for it. One of my patients had terrible sweats and pulmonary nodules. After an extensive evaluation I was still unable to secure a diagnosis. I suggested a PET scan, which, after I shouted and screamed, they finally approved — but they still would not guarantee payment. It is a $2000 test. The patient would not go, concerned that she might end up having to pay for it. Her diagnosis remained unresolved.

COUNTERPOINT: What is the name of these games? Why not just be forthright and honest? If we have the wrong code, tell us what the right one is. If you approve a test, do not say that you may not pay for it later. Do not leave a patient, who is already paying enormous premiums, holding the bag. Do not give our patients huge additional bills to pay, especially while you are already making massive profits. We are just trying to treat our patients. Could you please help us?

POINT: I ordered a bone markers test on a patient with worsening osteoporosis. This test is used all the time when pharmaceutical companies are studying the efficacy of their osteoporosis medications. I ordered this test very infrequently, but there were occasions when I felt that it could be clinically useful, especially for complicated cases of osteoporosis. For example, was this person's osteoporosis getting worse because the medication was not working or because she was not absorbing it properly or because she was not even taking it? The insurance company considered this test experimental, even though Medicare approves it. They refused my claim, and left the patient to pay for it.

COUNTERPOINT: So, I had to get on the phone and discuss the case with the insurance company's medical directors, one of whom was a general surgeon and the other a family practitioner. Neither knew anything about what this test is or how it might be used. After taking even more of my time to educate these two doctors about a test that they should at least have understood before they denied it, they finally approved it — just this one time. Hallelujah! Maybe they had thought that I would not pursue the situation, that they could just bill the patient for the test, and would collect her money without having to shell out any of their own.

In a similar situation I ordered a testosterone level test on a middle-aged male patient who complained of erectile dysfunction (ED). I had ordered this standard endocrinology test hundreds if not thousands of times previously without hassle from any insurance company. But this one time, this particular insurance company did not cover it. The patient was stuck with the $250 bill. After jumping through all their phone hoops, then using my gym voice to all their personnel who dared to get on the phone with me before they finally connected me to the head of the company, I got the test approved. My point? How could I, or any doctor, possibly know which companies would cover which medications or which tests before we ordered them? Do we have either the time or the energy to keep current with all the various insurance companies' catalogues to know which tests or meds are covered to what extent by which companies? They change their minds at the drop of a hat anyway. Is there no way to simplify the system?

POINT: The insurance company will only cover six Viagra per month.

COUNTERPOINT: This might be semi-legitimate, because they use the national average for the frequency of men having sex to determine how many Viagra tablets should be allowed each month. I only bring this example up to point out how dictatorial and in command the insurance companies are. Not only do they control most of the money and have most of the power, they also even tell our patients how often they can have sex each month.

Mulder's November 5, 2007, front-page article in the Syracuse *Post-Standard* was "Doctors Spar with Excellus over MRIs." He described the frustration that a local orthopedic surgeon, Dr. Irving G. Raphael, had with Excellus, the largest regional insurance company, in ordering an MRI scan for a female high school athlete to determine if she had a stress fracture and whether she could return to playing. Excellus denied the request, unless the surgeon could prove that the patient had a stress fracture first. But that was the point. He could not prove that she had a stress fracture and that was why he had ordered the MRI to begin with. Because Excellus would not approve the orthopedist's request for the MRI, he could not medically clear her to return to the playing field and she therefore missed her season.

To add salt to the physicians' and patients' wounds, Excellus put in place another hurdle for physicians to jump through to obtain MRI scans and other imaging studies for their patients, because Excellus thought that physicians were ordering too many scans. Excellus hired a company called CareCore National, that specializes in managing (limiting?) radiology utilization. This created an additional time and expense burden for physicians and their staffs. CareCore's staff would query each physician's staff, once we were able to get them on the phone, regarding reasons for each test, each patient's symptoms, last lab test, and other information. This process would take ten to fifteen minutes to complete. Mulder quoted Dr. Nancy Blake, "It's insulting that an insurance company is saying we physicians are not appropriately diagnosing and treating and we need their nurses' permission to order a CT scan."

If you do not yet have the picture, just do what I did: an informal survey. Ask the next ten fee-for-service doctors that you meet whether they have any frustrations or challenges in dealing with insurance companies. Ask whether the doctors even trust them. I would be surprised if the results were less than 100 per cent yes to the first question and no to the second. Ask them for examples too. I am sure that they would be happy to share a few with you. This conversation might be therapeutic for the doctors as well. You may actually be doing them a favor. Venting feels good.

The Only Trust is Mistrust

I have always felt that actions speak louder than words. My kids would sometimes say, when watching other kids play a sport, I can do that. My response would always be, "Show me." During my basketball playing days, I enjoyed the trash talking part of the game. When an opposing player said to me, "I'm going to score on you," I would always say, "Show me." Well, the insurance companies certainly showed me, with their actions, that they do not trust us physicians. Their actions were louder than any words. My first rule of any successful relationship is there has to be trust.

If I wanted to order any medication or test, I would have to fill out a preauthorization form or have my nurses contact the appropriate insurance company by phone, if they could get through, to get approval. Evidently, for the insurance companies, my years of study, training, and practicing medicine were not good enough. I apparently was not as qualified as they were to order medications or tests. I had to have their approval for my patient care decisions.

Sometimes an insurance company would want more information before approving my request. That is when I would get a letter with the two-word phrase that I came to loathe, "medical necessity." The insurance company would expect me to take time, which I did not have, and spend additional money, which I also did not have, to dictate a formal letter, have it transcribed, and send it to them, describing why I thought that the patient should have whatever test I was requesting and why I thought that their company should grant my request. It just was not good enough for them that a physician had ordered the medication or test. I certainly was not getting any kickback from ordering MRIs or PET scans. My only motivation was to treat my patients the best way I knew. Still, I had to justify to insurers, with my time and money, why I believed that these tests or meds were "medically necessary."

As I considered myself a patient advocate, I sent out those letters of medical necessity. I hoped that my requests would not be rejected for being what they considered, after conspiring with their paid medical directors, "medically unnecessary," experimental, or off-label indications. I half expected them to demand that I give them one of my children to get their approval — which I might actually have been willing to consider when my kids were teenagers. In the last paragraph of each of my letters of medical necessity, I asked the insurance company to reimburse me for the time and money that I had spent preparing the letter. As you may imagine, I received nothing in return. By the time I was ready to leave practice, frustrated, my letters of medical necessity would read as follows, "Because I said so ..."

Because they did not trust my ability or, evidently, my integrity, to send them the correct bill for whatever services I provided, they would periodically send "their team" to review my charts, i.e., to make sure that the billing code I submitted matched the work I did. When they received a bill, they would frequently, intentionally hold up payment, claiming that they needed more information, or that the diagnosis did not match the symptoms, or maybe for no particular reason at all.

Such insurance company actions have led to significant mistrust between physicians and insurance companies. Physicians have viewed these intrusions as assaults on our autonomy and integrity, two things that most physicians hold near and dear. They do not trust us. We, with justification, do not trust them. Consider these examples of the erosion of physicians' trust in insurance companies:

After years of medical societies and individual physicians complaining, UnitedHealthcare (UHC), one of the largest insurance companies in our country, was found in 2007 to have violated the laws of thirty-six states and the District of Columbia regarding claims payments. UHC was not paying for physician services in any timely manner, leaving us physicians with less money to pay bills promptly. UHC agreed to a multi-state settlement of twelve million dollars. It would thereafter need to meet or exceed strict benchmarks for claims processing: ninety-six per cent in 2008, ninety-seven in 2009 and 2010. But physicians got none of that twelve million. It all went to state insurance regulatory departments.

Insurance companies are exempt from antitrust laws. Even though individual insurance companies compete with each other, they are still all on the same team against us, my team. To that end, they can conspire with each other about economic issues, knowing full well that it is against the law for physicians to organize, to discuss fees, or to fix contracts. Thus the insurance companies can apply predatory pricing and manipulate their markets with little resistance.

The federal government vigorously prosecutes physicians who try to fight back, organize, and fix prices in contract negotiations with insurance companies. For example, Tanya Albert reported on January 12, 2004, in *amednews.com*, "The Newspaper for America's Physicians" at the AMA Web site <www.ama-assn.org/amednews/>, that six federal antitrust cases had been successful since 2002 against thousands of physicians from Maine to California, notably against a not-for-profit group of about 3000 in Houston, who had banded together to fight managed care. The federal commission claimed that their actions would have increased patient costs! These physicians were damned if they did and damned if they did not.

Insurance companies have begun to implement physician rating systems and to tell their patient subscribers which physicians are most cost-efficient — i.e., which physicians do not spend a lot of the insurance companies' money. These systems use medical billing data to rank physician efficiency and costs. There are several problems: First, the insurance companies do not routinely discuss cases with the involved physician and thus do not know the details of cases or the reasons why a physician might order certain medications or tests for particular patients. Second, a physician's rank is downgraded when patients do not comply with the physician's orders. Third, there may be clerical errors in the way that the companies collect the data, which can adversely affect a physician's rating. The companies' major concern is that some doctors, relative to their peers, may be ordering too many tests or medications, i.e., spending too much of the companies' money. The data that these companies collect, whether accurate or not, is then made available to the public, just like a baseball player's batting average or a quarterback's completion percentage. We may well ask whether a doctor who spends more money relative to his peers, and thus is deemed not cost-efficient, is bad for the patients or just for the insurance companies.

Every six months I received a Physician's Prescribing Report from Medco, the pharmacy benefit manager for one in four Americans. My last report looked at my prescribing habits, compared with my peers, from January 1 to June 30, 2007. During that time I wrote more total prescriptions and more prescriptions per Medco member (patient) than my peers did. I scrutinized Medco's data to try to see where the discrepancy lay. The answer was that I prescribed more cholesterol lowering and more blood pressure lowering medications. I spent more of the insurance companies' and Medco's money, but is that bad?

It is well documented that sixy to seventy per cent of people with diabetes will die from a heart attack or stroke. Their rate of such death is two to four times higher than that of the general population. People with diabetes live seven years less than the average American. It is also well documented that lowering cholesterol and blood pressure in diabetic people reduces their risk of coronary and cerebral vascular disease. Preventing myocardial infarctions and cerebral vascular accidents is much cheaper than treating them when they occur. So, although I spent more money on the front end, an impartial, rational person would think that my paying attention to these medical management details should be rewarded, not criticized. Data from the CDC National Center for Health Statistics (NCHS) National Health and Nutritional Examination Survey (NHANES), analyzed in 2004 by the National Diabetes Information Clearinghouse <diabetes.niddk.nih.gov/about/dateline/spr04/1.htm> and published in the *Diabetes Monitor* <www.diabetesmonitor.com/b322.htm>, showed that as of 2000 less than twelve per cent of diabetic adults had their blood sugars, blood pressure, and cholesterol at combined levels that met ADA standards, despite better understanding of the pathophysiology of diabetes and better treatments. I believe that, through my efforts and their compliance, at least fifty per cent my patients were either at or better than the ADA goal for these three important variables. But at what cost to the insurance companies? How did the insurers view their quarterly profits versus the long-term health of my patients?

I respect that insurance companies and even patients want data on physician performance, much like product information from *Consumer Guide* or *Consumer Reports*. It would be ideal if we could follow a physician's or a hospital's care by looking at the standings each day, how many patients lived and how many died, much like we would follow our favorite sports team in the print or online media. However, unlike in sports, where who won, who lost, who is at the top of the standings, and who is in the cellar, are all obvious and indisputable, determining quality or achievement in the game of medicine is not nearly as easy.

All my patients asked me who was the best endocrinologist they could go to after my practice closed. Sadly, I informed them, that there was no game, like the Super Bowl, a survivor show, *American Idol*, or *Dancing with the Stars*, which could determine who was the best doctor. The closest that we could get in making the analogy between sports and medicine would be ice skating or gymnastics, where judges, rather subjectively, would decide who was the best and who was not.

Obtaining and interpreting data as to who is the finest physician or which is the most excellent hospital is, at best, crude. Joe Rojas-Burke of the Newhouse News Service, in an article called "Health Care Ratings Challenge Consumers" that appeared in the January 7, 2008, Syracuse *Post-Standard*, cited a UCLA survey which showed that two different private companies hired to assess hospital surgery departments rated two of them as excellent while another private company rated the same two as poor. Rojas-Burke also cited a 2003 Case Western Reserve University study which revealed that prospective patients do not avoid hospitals with high death rates.

In my town, Syracuse, one hospital has a noticeably lower success rate for coronary bypass surgery than the other local hospitals. But these statistics are thought to be marred by the fact that this hospital operates on people who are sicker with more advanced disease.

Surveys over the years have consistently found, and anecdotes have often told, that most people prefer the advice of people they know and trust, such as their personal physicians, family members, or friends, instead of published data, even authoritative published data, that tries to show which physicians or hospitals are best.

Insurance companies and even the government have tried to undermine the most sacred of trusts, that between the physician and patient. Medicare has sent instructions to patients for turning their doctors in if the patients believe that the doctors bill fraudulently. I admit that some minority of physicians do commit fraud and should be found out and prosecuted. They certainly ruin things for the rest of us.

In the *Los Angeles Times* of February 28, 2008, surgeon SreyRam Kuy urged resistance against Blue Cross of California, which was asking physicians to report patients' conditions that could be used to cancel those patients' insurance. The California Medical Association responded to the crisis with a letter to state regulators protesting the idea of teammate spying on teammate. Blue Cross then curtailed its physician policing. That any insurance company would solicit help from its opponents, the physicians, to help with something that insurance companies are so good at already, i.e., cancelling patients' coverage, amazes me. Have they no shame? They cancel insurance policies for any reason at all, sometimes even for trivial, meanspirited reasons, like patients not filling out their forms correctly. They refuse to insure people with advanced medical problems, the ones who need insurance most, because such people would adversely affect the insurance companies' bottom lines.

Because fewer employers offer insurance coverage in 2009, some people go into the individual market to obtain health care, the market of last resort. The Commonwealth Fund reported on September 14, 2006, in a study called "Nearly Nine of Ten Who Seek Individual Market Health Insurance Never Buy a Plan" that fifty-eight per cent of 4000 surveyed working-age U.S. residents who were seeking individual health insurance found it unaffordable and that twenty-one per cent of these 4000 were either rejected, charged higher premiums, or offered policies that excluded coverage for their particular health conditions. Syndicated columnist Susan Estrich wrote sarcastically in a May 7, 2008, editorial that Republican presidential candidate John McCain would have been turned down from his own proposed health care plan because of his age, over seventy, and his pre-existing conditions, including cancer and major surgery. Even with all his wife's money, the individual insurers likely still would not have covered him.

In many respects, the insurance companies have become the general manager, or maybe even the boss, of "my team": the patients, their employers, and the physicians. I believe that most physicians resent this. The insurers have usurped economic power, control, and trust. They evidently expect that we will follow their orders and play according to their rules. But, they may be wrong.

President Eisenhower said at a news conference on August 4, 1954: "A platoon leader doesn't get his platoon to go by getting up and shouting and saying, 'I am smarter, I am bigger, I am stronger, I am the leader.' He gets men to go along with him because they want to do it for him and they believe in him." Great leaders lead by example, not by command. Thus the idea that physicians would ever follow the insurance companies, like good soldiers, is farfetched. Rather, physicians feel bullied by insurance companies.

Some physicians may be trying to fight back, or trying to add extra oomph to their counterpunches, by joining unions. They would thus risk antitrust violations, as lawyer Elinor R. Hoffmann suggested in "Physicians' Unions: Handle With Care" <library.findlaw.com/1998/Mar/1/127470.html>. How many physicians in America are actually members of unions? Who knows? American physician unionization has reached only the blogging stage, such as Joshua Micah Marshall's "Talking Points Memo," "The TPM Blog": <tpmcafe.talkingpointsmemo. com/talk/blogs/tmcpac/2009/03/why-health-insurance-companies-1.php>.

They Make More and There Are More of Them

The December 27, 2007, front-page headline of the Syracuse *Post-Standard* was "CEO Said 'No' to Riches." The CEO was Howard Berman, who had retired from Excellus in 2004. Mulder described how Berman had renounced the tens of millions that he could have made by converting the company from not-for-profit to for-profit. When asked why he did not take this money he just said, "It would be wrong." Many other CEOs in the same position did not have the same conscience. But he apparently felt that accepting a three-year retirement package of 1.69 million dollars in 2004 and 1.74 million in both 2005 and 2006 was not wrong.

Mulder's article, essentially a feature book review of Johnston's *Free Lunch*, cited several passages from that book, including:

What Berman saw was that shifting from an enterprise whose purpose was to serve people into a for-profit business would mean something worse than enriching the few at the expense of the many. It would also, inevitably, mean getting rich at the expense of people's health, not their betterment ... spending a smaller share of health care premiums on actual care. If health care as a business worked, it would be a success story to embrace. ... We pay more, enjoy shorter lives, and are drowning in infuriating make-work, filing claims and making appeals, while distorting the whole economy because one giant component is a commercial activity. No other modern country regards health care as an insurance business.

Berman was the exception, not the rule. Johnston described in *Free Lunch* how Leonard Schaeffer made over 100 million dollars by converting California Blue Cross into WellPoint in 1986. Similar profits accrued to Fred Wasserman and Pamela Anderson when they converted not-for-profit Maxicare of California into a for-profit company, and to Robert Gumbiner, who converted the HMO he had founded for the poor into a for-profit company. Gumbiner's shares were worth 115 million dollars. Virginia's not-for-profit Blue Shield / Blue Cross paid its CEO under $900,000 in 1995, but in 2001, after becoming for-profit, its CEO made 6.5 million dollars in salary and sixteen million in stock options. Those extra dollars could have been spent on delivering health care.

The not-for-profit CEOs are not doing too badly either. *The Buffalo News* reported on July 8, 2007, in "Here's What Health Insurers Pay Top Execs," that the combined take-home pay of the three CEOs of the three largest New York State not-for-profit health insurance companies was 3.77 million dollars in 2006. Meanwhile, employers' health insurance premiums had increased for employees each year since 1996 (up 5.3 per cent in 1999, 8.2 per cent in 2000, 10.9 per cent in 2001, 12.9 per cent in 2002, 13.9 per cent in 2003, 11.2 per cent in 2004, and 9.2 per cent in 2005, according to Kaiser Family Foundation data. Kaiser also said that these premiums had gone up a total of seventy-three per cent from

2000 to 2005. Dr. Thomas A. Bersani, then President of the Onondaga County Medical Society, published a letter to the editor of the Syracuse *Post-Standard* on December 27, 2007, stating that health insurance policy holders in the Syracuse area paid fifty-one per cent more in 2007 than in 2003, "despite the fact that our health care costs here are among the lowest in the country and Syracuse has ... the lowest hospital utilization rates in the State." Where is all this money going? It is not hard to figure that out.

In 2006 Excellus, the largest not-for-profit in Upstate New York, paid its CEO 1.78 million dollars, its vice chairman 1.75 million, and its senior vice president and CFO 1.48 million. It paid 10.3 million dollars to its top ten officers and another forty million to 250 others who made over $100,000 each. The company's overhead was another 253 million. That was 300 million spent on just administering health care. Those extra dollars too could have been spent on delivering health care. The for-profits are worse.

Examining the financial compensation of for-profit health insurance company CEOs brings to mind words like lavish, exorbitant, excessive, obscene, and ridiculous. The average compensation for the highest paid executives of the eleven leading health care companies in 2002, according to "Top Dollar: CEO Compensation in Medicare's Private Insurance Plans," the June 2003 Families USA report <www.familiesusa.org/assets/pdfs/Top_Dollar_report.pdf>, was 15.1 million dollars. Norman Payson of Oxford Health Plans took the most, a staggering seventy-six million dollars per year. But that is chump change compared with the unexercised stock options of these top executives, the average being 67.7 million, and the top being UnitedHealth's McGuire at 529.9 million! Again, all those extra dollars could have been spent on actually delivering health care.

David Whelan's "This Won't Hurt a Bit: No Company Benefits More than WellPoint from the Current Health Care Mess" in the September 17, 2007, *Forbes* highlighted Well-Point's CEO, Angela Braly, "the most powerful woman in health care," and sixteenth on the Forbes list of the World's Most Powerful Women. Why? Even pro-capitalist *Forbes* did not shy away from testifying to the coldness that lies under her warm exterior. In 2006 WellPoint had sales of fifty-six billion dollars. Its earnings rose fifty-five per cent each year since 2000 to three billion in 2006. Its revenues grew thirty-seven per cent each year in that same period. Its premium growth rate (PGR) significantly exceeds the consumer price index (CPI). For all this Braly gets 2.8 million dollars in annual salary, bonuses, and stock options. But what do patients and doctors get? At least ten patients sued, but settled out of court their claims that WellPoint had unfairly cancelled their policies. Class action lawsuits from physicians have alleged that WellPoint withholds payments. WellPoint has spent two million of its hard-earned dollars attacking California Governor Arnold Schwarzenegger's plan to provide health insurance for everyone. David Colby, the CFO who had competed with Braly for the CEO position before she was hired, was fired by WellPoint because of personal misconduct, i.e., dating twelve women at once including a WellPoint employee who was suing the company. He left with a paltry 180 million dollars in stock. That money could have bought 18,000 families $10,000 worth of health insurance each.

The *Boston Globe* reported on January 27, 2007, that Massachusetts adds to the pain and suffering of the people who pay health insurance premiums by paying the administrators who oversee the state's universally mandated insurance plan over six figures each. These ordinary citizens, who likely could not afford insurance to begin with (otherwise they may not have had to be mandated to buy it) have the cost of these executives' salaries passed on to them by the insurers, who now charge the Massachusetts government a four to five per cent surcharge. Just when you think you might crumble under such staggering numbers, the news seems to get worse. Higher health insurance premiums each year are beginning to seem as inevitable as death and taxes.

PNHP and other proponents of a not-for-profit, governmental, single-payer system guesstimate that around 300 *billion* dollars could be saved each year just by the natural simplifying of administration. Those savings alone would insure all forty-seven million uninsured in America and upgrade coverage for the rest of us. Steffie Woolhandler *et al.* in the August 21, 2003, *NEJM* argued that the U.S. system could markedly reduce administrative costs if it more closely resemble Canada's.

Good Patients Do Not Leave Good Doctors (Unless Their Insurance Changes)

Patients sometimes left my practice feeling that they were not receiving the type of advice or care they sought. At first, I was saddened by them leaving. I felt like I had let them down and should have done more. But, as time wore on, I was happy that some of those patients had left, because there was no way that I could satisfy their needs or demands. Take Ms. M., a young woman from a town about forty-five minutes from Syracuse. She had hyperthyroidism and its associated depression and anxiety disorder. I spent endless hours with her and her husband, both in the office and on the phone, discussing her condition and the different treatment options available. I helped to regulate her thyroid with medications, which allowed her to conceive. During her pregnancy, I followed her even more closely, if possible, to try to ensure a good outcome.

After she delivered her child she finally decided to take radioactive iodine for her thyroid. My office made all the arrangements and she had the treatment uneventfully. As expected, she developed hypothyroidism, which I treated. Nevertheless, whenever she did not feel well, even for a day, she blamed her thyroid, although her thyroid blood tests were optimal. Try as I may, I could not convince her otherwise. She believed that she would not feel well until we fixed what was broken.

The last straw for her came when she had thyroid blood tests done only a few days apart. Usually these tests are measured, at minimum, weeks apart, because thyroid numbers change very slowly. There was one change in the thyroid result that I considered negligible, a lab variation, but she considered significant. As bad luck would have it, the Friday that her test came back was the one day in over sixteen years of practice that I was too sick to come into work, though I tried, even crawling to my bedroom door only to be rebuffed by my caring wife. That day gave me newfound respect for the concept of vomiting.

When I felt better, Sunday night, I called her from my home to review the tests, because she had made an angry call to my staff the day I was out. That night she informed me that she was going to another doctor who would listen to her complaints and not blow her off. I have been called many things by many people, but, despite treating tens of thousands of people over my medical career, none of them ever told me that I was not a good listener. In fact, I prided myself on this. But for Ms. M., it just was not good enough. Although I initially regretted her leaving my practice, given all the time and effort that I had put into her care, in the end I felt relieved as I recalled the physicians' adage, "Good patients don't leave good doctors."

However, in our health care environment in the early twenty-first century, that adage no longer held true. Many good patients over the years were forced to leave my practice because of the insurance debacle affecting our whole country.

For example, when I left my hospital-based practice in 2004 to join FPA, hundreds of patients could not come with me to the new practice because FPA did not accept their Empire insurance plan. Why not? Because every time FPA saw an Empire patient, it lost money. Again, none of us were in the medical field to strike it rich, but we did not expect to have to lose money either.

When I transferred my practice to FPA, we called the executives at the Empire plan and told them of our predicament. We asked them to raise the reimbursement rate so that at least we would not be seeing each patient for a loss. We told Empire that otherwise we would have to let all those patients go, leaving them to scramble to find other endocrinology care. We reminded Empire that I had already established rapport and trust with these patients and that there was a shortage of endocrinologists in our area. Empire's callous, coldhearted response was, "Have the patients find other care." Money trumped the doctor/patient relationship again.

I have also been on the receiving end of such circumstances. A patient came to me from another endocrinologist's practice, where he had been receiving excellent care for over fifteen years. He trusted that doctor's opinions, and the doctor knew his history backwards and forwards, as well as his likes and dislikes. But, only because of insurance, that patient had to leave a comfortable, pleasant, trusting medical situation to re-establish it all over again. My mother had always implored me to look at each state of affairs from all sides, but it was just hard to digest that money ever matters more than people and their relationships.

There were also good patients who left my practice because they lost their jobs and the insurance that went along with it. Not only do we estimate that the number of uninsured people increases by one million for every one per cent increase in the national unemployment rate, but also that the number of people on Medicaid or the State Children's Health Insurance Program (SCHIP) likewise increases by one million.

We were always willing to work with patients when they were between jobs, developing reasonable payment plans for them, like paying us maybe $10 a month. But eventually their bills became so overwhelming that such patients just decided that they could not afford any medical care and just did without it. People have pride. It embarrassed them that they owed so much money and that I was still willing to continue to treat them as if they all had gold cards. I would have treated them for free. But I had no financial cushion either. Our practice was in the red each month and eventually it succumbed to financial shortfall.

When those lost patients found other jobs and came back to the practice, we had to start all over again getting them back on their medical regimens, because they had stopped not only going to the doctor, but also taking their medications. So, when they came back, their sugars, blood pressures, and cholesterol numbers were off the wall and their risk of disease complications was even greater, potentially costing the system even more money. The old saying, "Penny wise, pound foolish," came quickly to mind.

"Give Us Our Profession Back! (or Maybe We'll Just Take It)"

The insurance companies make up rules and regulations, without physician input, that seem to benefit only them, especially financially. Then they expect us, the physicians, to play by those made-up rules. They are like malevolent shepherds. We are the sheep that they push in directions that we do not want to go. They make us act in ways that we do not want to act. How can that be fair? Somehow — but probably as a development from President Nixon's concessions to Kaiser Permanente in 1973 that led to the formation of HMOs — the insurance companies have hijacked the health care system, taken almost complete control of medical finances, and usurped actual medical decisions. How could we have allowed this to happen?

My dentist friends call me an "RD," a "real doctor." However, given that the insurance companies have taken over the medical profession, dentists must now think that this "RD" stands for "really dumb." How were dentists able to be smart enough not to get themselves into an analogous predicament? When I go to my dentist he does whatever he wants, and at the end of the visit I pay him whatever he charges me. There are no preauthorizations to fill out, no staff sitting on the phone waiting to talk with any insurance company personnel, and no letters that the dentist needs to send to any insurance company to justify that his treatment is "dentally necessary." He never worries that one of his claims will be rejected or that payments will be delayed.

National medical societies, like the AMA and the American College of Physicians (ACP), and even some local medical societies, are desperately trying to fight, to become our saviors. They represent us with bright, caring, articulate physicians, who dedicate significant amounts of their personal time, often after office hours, to struggle against the insurance companies and government mandates. We appear to be, however, always on the reactive, never proactive. It seems that the insurance companies and government always have us backpedaling, forcing us, the providers, to react to their decisions. Why is that? Why not have them backpedal? Why do we not just declare that this is what we doctors have decided about our patients and that you non-medical people, who do not even know our patients, should not be spending your time and efforts countering our clinical recommendations? Why is there any backpedalling by anyone? Are we not all in this together?

Insurance company CEOs and top executives are making, taking, not earning, more than ever with enormous salaries and stock options. What makes this grasping even more unpalatable is that they generate their incomes from our efforts to deliver medical care. Even more distressing is that they make more money when they deny care rather than allow it to be provided.

Insurance companies have hired medical doctors to help them dominate the medical profession. These physicians seem to be mercenaries, and at the very least have significant conflicts of interest. Even though they are physicians, and are thus supposed to be concerned first with patients' health and welfare, they are paid bonuses for denying tests and treatments that we have ordered for our patients. Maybe this problem was best articulated by Dr. J.S. Hochman, executive director of the National Foundation for the Treatment of Pain, in "Insurance and Healthcare: An Irresolvable Conflict" at <www.paincare.org/about/message.php?id=361>: "Typically the financial compensation to these 'Medical Directors' is directly tied to the number of denials they generate. As many of these Medical Directors have revealed, after leaving employment with insurers, the job is morally corrupt, professionally unacceptable as physicians, personally demoralizing, and an irresolvable conflict with their most profound duties as doctors. The management of insurance companies, almost universally non-physicians, has no such perceptible conflicts. This fiction of 'medical review', removes the management of insurance companies from much of the direct responsibility for the denial of care. Their captive physicians, nurses and pharmacists do it.."

What about the physicians who work for the insurance industry? How do they rationalize their relationship with the "other team?"

Dr. Linda Peeno, former medical claims reviewer for Humana, former HMO medical director, former hospital medical director, and former physician executive for Blue Cross / Blue Shield of Kentucky, testified before the U.S. House of Representatives on May 30, 1996. Her testimony, available online at <www.thenationalcoalition.org/DrPeenotestimony.html>, exemplified Dr. Hochman's message. She said in her confession to the legislature that she had killed a man just by doing what her company expected of her, using her medical expertise to deny him care, and, in the process, saved the company $500,000. She stated that "managed care is inherently unethical in the areas of both medicine and business," and that her experiences were "standard practice and quite ordinary for the managed care business." Dr. Peeno rejoined "our team" and is now a medical ethics consultant and a managed care watchdog.

Robert P. Gervais, M.D., an Arizona ophthalmologist, echoed Peeno's and Hochman's sentiments in "Managed Care Is Inherently Unethical and Should Be Scuttled," published in volume 4 of the *Medical Sentinel* (1999) <www.jpands.org/hacienda/gervais1.html>.

If the insurance companies' goals are to wear us down, then they are very successful. Who has the time, energy, or patience to sit on the phone only to have a claim or test rejected — by a non-medical person? The only people I have ever yelled at were my kids — only when necessary, of course — and various insurance company personnel. Like many of my colleagues, who are usually mild-mannered, calm, cool, and collected, I became so exasperated with the steeplechase that the insurers made my staff and I run each day just to get things done that, I am embarrassed to say, I even used expletives ... frequently. They push us all to our limits of tolerance and composure.

I remain confused as to what value the insurance companies bring to the care of our patients, especially given their significant self-compensation. I am always amazed that they claim to know what is best for our patients, whom they never see, talk to, or examine. How can they do that and yet have no liability issues?! They can fix prices, but, if physicians ever tried to do so, it would violate the antitrust laws. Doctors have become so frustrated that we have even started to join unions. What's next, a strike? Concierge or boutique practices that eliminate the insurance companies' influence on physicians but further limit the people's access to medical care?

Physicians tend to be altruistic. The insurers take advantage of our good-naturedness. They use our patients as human shields for their skulduggery, knowing how deeply committed we are to them.

Each year patients' premiums increase and business owners' health care costs go up, in spite of the insurance companies' millions and billions of dollars in reserve. Each year many of our patients complained more and felt like they got less for their money. Did you ever try to read through the details of health insurance policies? Could they ever make it any more complicated? Thank goodness that my wife is a lawyer who could help to try to decipher the fine print. What do people do who do not have such easy access to an attorney to guide them through these convoluted, confusing health insurance contracts?

When HMOs became popular in the 1990s, their goal was to improve the quality of health care while keeping expenses down. But since then, health care costs have dramatically outpaced inflation and the profits of these companies have soared. They even offered physicians opportunities to participate in capitated systems in which the docs would take on both the medical and the financial liabilities of the patients. What a scheme that was! This idea would have put us in significant conflict of interest with our patients. The insurance companies would give the physicians a fixed amount of money to spend on each patient each year. If the doctors spent all this allotment ordering tests or seeing patients in the office, they would lose money. If, on the other hand, the doctors ordered fewer tests or saw patients less frequently, they would make money. The *fewer* tests and office visits, the more money the doctors would make! Doctors would make more money by offering *less* care to patients. Could you believe this heartless idea? I vehemently opposed the arrangement.

Doctors resent their loss of freedom and independence. I believe that the field of medicine attracts people who like to think for themselves and appreciate autonomy. Many of us went into medicine with the idea that we would review the literature and use our scientific acumen and clinical experience to best treat our patients. We feel that our independence has been stripped away. We have to jump through the insurers' preauthorization hoops for tests, referrals, and certain medications. These requirements mean employing more staff and using more of their time, thereby increasing our expenses without improving patient care. They not only put up such obstacles to efficient patient care, but each insurance company — and there are many of them — has its own unique and arbitrary set of rules. How can we remember all those different rules and policies? Would it not be better to have just one set of insurance rules, generated by physicians and based upon medical evidence, or just reasonable care, to order tests and medicines? We feel that we need to ask permission from the insurance companies' non-medical personnel whenever we want to use our trained judgment or do what we believe is medically right for our patients. It reminds me of the credit card commercial where the answer to any request is simply "NO!"

I suspect that the only people who are happy with our health care system are those few who are fully insured, are receiving adequate care and are thus understandably afraid of any change in the system, or are financially profiting from the system. There appears to be no motivation for the people in power, the insurance companies, the pharmaceutical industry, or the politicians who enjoy financial benefit via lobbyists, to change our "free market system" — which is certainly not "free" for the patients or employers who are forced to accommodate increasing premiums each year. While we doctors evaluate people, the "other team" evaluates profits. For them, money matters most. For us, people matter most. We need to have a system that is best for most, not just for the select fortunate few.

The American system has made the physicians' hard job even harder. My daily mantra to survive was, "I'm doing the best I can." Some days were so difficult that I was not sure if I could answer the bell the next day. Mondays were of course the hardest days, because patients, having saved their problems from Saturday and Sunday, seemed to call all at once. My Monday night mantra, trying to keep myself positive, was, "Tomorrow will be better ..."

What a difference a day made, or three or four days, because by Friday afternoon I would rationalize and say, "It wasn't that bad." I would take good naps both Saturday and Sunday afternoons. By Sunday evening I would start feeling normal again, only to have Monday come again. Those days are now behind me, but continue to exist for my brothers and sisters still practicing medicine and for the patients trying to survive this onerous system.

It is hard for physicians to deliver optimal medical care when we feel demoralized and dispirited. My colleagues and I, who are usually mild-mannered, kind, caring, and altruistic, have suffered too many unfair decisions and lopsided defeats against our rival, the insurance companies. Our job demands that we concentrate and focus, that we be fresh for each patient encounter, and that we always present ourselves as compassionate and empathetic. Michael Jordan could dunk a basketball just once and everyone would see it at the same instant. He was allowed to miss a few shots. But we physicians have to make a slam dunk each and every time, at least twenty to thirty times each day, with each individual patient. We cannot miss a shot. Feeling oppressed and constantly pressured by the system in which we must operate makes achieving our goals more difficult. Unfortunately, for many physicians, the aggravation of practicing medicine is exceeding the satisfaction. I have left already and more physicians are considering it: "We can't hold it in anymore."

Chapter Fourteen

The Pharmaceutical Industry

Marketing Budgets Trump Research and Development Budgets Any Day

"You can keep the pens, pads, and even the lunch," I said to test the young and attractive pharmaceutical representative. "Let's get serious about advertising. See my white lab coat? I would like to make it look like a NASCAR racer. Our practice is losing money each month. We need the money to keep our practice open. I know that your company is flushed with money. How could it not be with the prices you are charging my patients for their medications. Let's make a deal. I'll sell your company a place on my lab coat and in return you get my endorsement. I'll even put your Viagra sign lower on my jacket, in the front, to give it the full meaning. That will save me room for Lipitor near my heart, Nexium near my gut, Celebrex on my arm between my shoulder and elbow, and Synthroid on my collar near my neck. There will still be room saved on my back for the bull's-eye for the malpractice attorneys and insurance companies to shoot at." Although I was (half) kidding, she seemed interested.

Each day while I was in practice I would be besieged by pharmaceutical salespeople telling me about the wonders of their drugs. They are not really salespeople. They are more like lobbyists, people who try to influence other people's behaviors. They knew that I did not actually buy anything that they were trying to sell. Rather, they hoped that I would feel comfortable with them and their products and, in turn, prescribe their medications for my patients, who would then become the buyers, sometimes at exorbitant prices, so that vast profits would return to their company. These representatives would be paid bonuses based upon how influential they had been in affecting doctors' behaviors; i.e., the more of their medications that were prescribed in their respective territories, the greater their bonuses.

These pharmaceutical reps were incredibly nice. Most were extremely good looking and many were smart. They are very good at what they were trained to do; after all, the companies that hired them are kings of marketing. These companies have spent considerable time and money figuring out how to sell their drugs. In fact, as Dr. Marcia Angell reports in *The Truth About the Drug Companies: How They Deceive Us and What to Do About It* (2005), despite the pharmaceutical companies' assertions, studies show that they spend more money on advertising than they do on research and development (R and D). Thus it is no wonder that, as she emphasizes in several ways, the top ten pharmaceutical companies continue to reap greater profits than the remainder of the Fortune 500 companies.

To influence us physicians, the pharmaceutical representatives brought us little *chatchkas* (the Yiddish word for "meaningless stuff"), which I considered *hazoray* (the Yiddish word for "junk"), and which almost always ended up in the circular file. They also gave, or mailed to us, product literature that looked very expensive to make, produced by studies that their companies sponsored. It barely touched my hands before I tossed it out like a hot potato. I was always suspicious that their medication studies were biased.

Biases similar to mine against pharmaceutical-sponsored drug studies were highlighted in "Impugning the Integrity of Medical Science: The Adverse Effects of Industry Influence," an editorial in *JAMA* by Catherine DeAngelis and Phil Fontanarosa, April 16, 2008. They described ghost writers who had been hired by for-profit information industries, but were then hired by different pharmaceutical companies to write scientific drug studies for publication. The pharmaceutical companies then would slap the names of highly regarded academicians onto the articles, after paying fees to these professors, even though they had little or nothing to do with the studies. *JAMA*'s additional concern was that the final publications may withhold, misrepresent, or tweak the actual scientific or clinical results to make the companies' medications look more favorable.

The pharmaceutical representatives would also, on occasion, sign up for a day of preceptorship, during which they would follow me around the office masquerading as students trying to learn what I do as a physician, so that they could better serve my needs and the needs of my patients. It was really a marketing ploy, a way for representatives to establish a quick relationship with me — they know that relationships sell products — and to advertise their products all day. What was in it for me? I was paid a three-figure honorarium for the day to mentor the novice.

In general, their strategies must work. They certainly spend a lot of money trying to influence physician behaviors, i.e., about seven billion dollars per year, a 275 per cent rise from 1996 to 2004, according to "Ties That Bind" by Barbara Basler in the *AARP Bulletin*, January-February 2008. Even if we deny it, I believe that many physicians are influenced by their strategies. I was.

Eric G. Campbell *et al.* reported in "A National Survey of Physician-Industry Relationships" in *NEJM*, April 26, 2007, that ninety-four per cent of physicians have direct ties to the pharmaceutical industry. This industry has done studies to show that, if a drug rep spends just one minute with a physician, then the doctor increases prescription writing for the promoted drug by about sixteen per cent. If the rep spends three minutes with the doc, then the prescription writing for that drug increases about fifty-two per cent. I admit that if there were several choices of the same medications that could help my patient — "me-too" drugs — and if they all cost and worked about the same, then I would choose the one drug that was represented by the pharmaceutical representative whom I liked the most. That is just human nature, and the pharmaceutical industry is well aware of it.

Like many physicians who understood the conflict of interest between the pharmaceutical industry and themselves, as Susan Chimonas *et al.* discussed in the February 2007 issue of the *Journal of General Internal Medicine*, I used some of my best defense mechanisms, like denials and rationalizations, so that I would not think that I was doing anything wrong. I allowed pharmaceutical representatives into my office for two main reasons, for better or worse: First, they brought "free" lunch. It was a perk for my staff to have a different lunch every day. I rationalized that, the happier the staff, the better they would work and — I hoped — the longer they would stay. Second, and equally important, the representatives brought us "free" samples of their medications, so that patients just starting a new medicine could try it before they purchased it. The pharmaceutical companies, I suspect, hoped that if one of my patients started one of their medicines, and if it worked without side effects, then the patient would be more likely to want to continue that medicine and pay for it. Of course, the samples were not "free." The pharmaceutical companies are not generous enough to give away eighteen billion dollars worth of samples each year. Yet this was the figure that Basler reports was determined in 2005 by the Prescription Project, funded by the Pew Charitable Trust. The costs of these samples were built into the price of each drug when the patients or their insurers eventually purchased it, as was each "free" lunch.

Yet there were some good reasons for me to have medication samples available. A patient feeling ready to start a new medication could begin it immediately. According to the March 2008 Harvard School of Public Health study, "The Public on Prescription Drugs and Pharmaceutical Companies," available online at <www.kff.org/kaiserpolls/upload/7748. pdf>: "Four in ten adults (41%) say it is at least somewhat of a problem for their family to pay for prescription drugs they need, including 16% who say it is a serious problem ... Three in ten (29%) say that in the last two years, they have not filled a prescription because of the cost, and nearly a quarter (23%) say they have cut pills in half or skipped doses in order to make a medication last longer." Such patients relied on medical offices, like mine, to supply them with free medications. If we did not have the samples, then they went without their meds and their conditions went untreated and sometimes got worse.

Even though this Harvard study said that only nineteen per cent of Americans take four or more medications each day, it was common for many of my patients to be on a double-digit number of medications, which is called polypharmacy. They had diabetes, high blood pressure, high cholesterol, heart disease, peripheral vascular disease, kidney disease, thyroid disease, arthritis, gastrointestinal reflux problems, as well as insomnia, anxiety, and depression — as who would not with all those problems and the need for all those medications? I felt that there should be a pill for every malady, as did the patients. I thought that it would be ideal, as some have proposed, to have just one pill, called a polypill, which would have all their medicines in one, even though the size of that pill could make it impossible to swallow. Never mind even thinking about taking it as a suppository.

Pitch to the Patients

Patients are bombarded with pharmaceutical advertisements on TV, in magazines, on the Internet, in grocery stores, as well as in pharmacies. Heck, you cannot even watch a baseball game anymore without Viagra, Levitra, or Cialis being in your face — whether between innings in the many commercials or between pitches in advertisements on the backstop behind the catcher. My kids were asking me questions about these drugs when they were adolescents, which hastened our discussion about the birds and the bees, not to mention introducing the word "condom" into our talks.

The goal of the pharmaceutical companies, via these direct-to-consumer (DTC) advertisements is to sell more medications by raising questions to the patients like, "Are you suffering from 'fecaloculitis,' ('a shitty outlook on life'), and, if you are, is this medication right for you? Sure it is. Now go ask your doctor to prescribe it, go on." Maybe the companies hoped that the doctor would think that the drug was a good idea and would thank the company for educating the patient. Or that the doctor would be too busy to think about the diagnosis. Or that the doc, being too worn out by everything else, would not fight with the patient about using that particular medication, but would just sigh and acquiesce. Does the DTC strategy work? You bet it does!

Ninety-one per cent of all Americans saw or heard prescription drug ads in 2008, according to the March 2008 Harvard study, up from eighty-one per cent in 2002 and seventy-two per cent in 1999, according to Food and Drug Administration (FDA) survey figures.

The 2004 FDA survey revealed that, in 2002, forty-three per cent of patients sought additional information about a medication after hearing or seeing a DTC ad, and that eighty-nine per cent of these seekers got this information from their doctors and fifty-one per cent from their pharmacists. As Elizabeth Murray *et al.* reported in the July-September 2003 issue of the *Journal of Medical Internet Research*, physicians are not enamored of patients bringing in information from the Internet. Many thought that it challenged their authority or made office visits less time-efficient. Again according to the March 2008 Harvard study, eighty-two per cent of the patients who talked to their doctor about an ad that they had seen got either the exact drug they requested or a comparable one. DTC ads work!

There are more DTC advertisements than ever, even though FDA data from 2004 shows that patients are enjoying these ads less and less. Thirty-two per cent of consumers liked them in 2002, down from fifty-two per cent in 1999. Despite this, FDA surveys consistently show that more drugs are prescribed now than ever before. Data collected in 2007 by Medco Health Solutions and reported on May 14, 2008, by the Associated Press revealed that fifty-one per cent of Americans were taking at least one medication for a chronic condition, up from forty-seven per cent in 2001, with the largest increase, twenty per cent, occurring in twenty-to-forty-four-year-olds, treating conditions like depression, diabetes, asthma, attention deficit disorder (ADD), and tendency to seizures. Moreover, also according to Medco, Americans buy more medications than any other people in the world.

I do not know how people swallow all those pills each day. Many do not. Patient non-compliance rate with medications in 2008 was about twenty-nine per cent in the U.S., according to Prof. Richard Hirth at the University of Michigan School of Public Health. I also do not know how people afford all those pills.

It is Expensive to Stay Alive

It seemed to me that the people who needed the most medications were often the ones who were least able to afford them, our seniors on fixed incomes and those with chronic diseases.

Even people with prescription plans had to pay a co-pay for each refill. Those refill co-pays added up fast and high for ten to fifteen different medications each month. People in the Medicare part D program also had financial challenges, especially if they were in the "donut hole," the built-in coverage gap.

Although, according to the March 2008 Harvard School of Public Health study, seventy-three per cent of Americans believe that drugs developed since the 1980s have made their lives better, forty-four per cent have unfavorable opinions of pharmaceutical companies, i.e., less favorable than either health insurance companies (fifty-four per cent) or oil companies (sixty-three per cent). Sixty-eight per cent say that their biggest gripe with the pharmaceutical industry is the prices that they have to pay for prescribed medications. People believe that these high prices are associated with the pharmaceutical industry's greed and high profits.

I was happy to be able to *shtup* (the Yiddish word for giving something to someone for nothing) my patients as many "free" medications as possible to keep them as well as possible. I knew that the medications were not really "free" and neither were the lunches. The patients who were actually buying the medications at full price were, in part, paying for our lunches and the medicines for the patients who could not afford them. On a grander scale, our population subsidizes the prescription drug purchases of the entire world. *Medical News Today* <www.medicalnewstoday.com/articles/93397.php> reported on January 9, 2008, that only Japan has higher drug prices, and that American drug prices range from six to thirty-three per cent higher than those in the rest of the world.

My practice was located in Central New York, about a ninety-mile drive to Canada. One of my elderly patients, on a fixed income, had a pituitary tumor producing excess prolactin, the milk hormone. He needed a medication called Dostinex, generically called cabergoline. It was much cheaper for him to drive 180 miles round trip to Canada, even with the increasing gas prices, and to risk getting caught at the border with "illegal" drugs, than to pay the ridiculously high price for the medication in his own country. I know that he is not alone. Patients who live far from Canada use the Internet to buy their medications from our northern neighbor. In June 2004 the

Council of State Governments <www.csg.org> reported that
seven American cities and thirteen American states had plans
to re-import medications from Canada to try to control their
skyrocketing health care costs for their public employees,
even though such transactions were still illegal.

I gave out as many "free" samples as possible, because
nothing could be as defeating to me as working very hard with
the patients to get them on exactly the right medical formula,
only to have them stop taking their medications or squirrel
them away, just taking them on occasion, simply to save money.
It was defeating to my patients, and to me, to see their diabetes, blood pressure, or cholesterol levels deteriorate after
having had them "at goal," just because they had stopped
taking their high-cost meds. Worse, their risk of negative and
expensive consequences of their medication noncompliance
would increase the cost of their health care even more.

I stopped asking patients if they were taking their medications. Rather, I asked them how often they were missing
them. If I asked a patient, "Are you taking your med?" the
answer would frequently be, "Yes." If I then said, "How
often are you taking it?" then I might hear, "A couple of
times a week." Then I would push harder, "But you said you
were taking it," to which the patient would say, "Yes, I am
taking the medication, but when you first asked me if I was
taking it, you didn't ask me how often." So, I stopped this
Abbott and Costello routine by asking them directly how
often they missed their medication each week, not whether
they were taking it. That way, if a patient's condition was
getting worse, I would know whether it was from being on
the wrong drug, having an inadequate dose of the right drug,
or not taking the drug adherently.

We Are Surrounded, but Beginning to Fight Back

What remains most distasteful to me about the pharma/phy-
sician relationship is that, in the end, it is the patients who suffer the most, both financially and medically. The company's
representatives flatter us with comments like, "Doctor, you
are a thought leader and we really trust your opinion about

this drug," then entice us with their *chatchkas* and lunches, all so that we will prescribe their expensive medications. But where does this leave the patients? Clearly, it burdens them with medical costs that many cannot afford, thus rendering their treatable medical conditions untreatable.

I admit that I was guilty of being involved in this deception of our patients as well. I am, to use another Yiddish word, no *tatala* ("good boy"). But I am not alone. Other physicians have faced the same dilemma. The reps must be doing a good job "selling" (pushing?) their medications; otherwise the companies would not hire so many of them.

Some physicians fight back against the influence that pharmaceutical companies impose on physicians. Web sites like "No Free Lunch" <www.nofreelunch.org/> and "Pharmed Out" <www.pharmedout.org/> are part of this fight. The IOM has been drawing up guidelines to reduce doctors' conflict of interest. Federal and state legislators have been trying to pass laws that would require pharmaceutical companies to report gifts to physicians of over $25 or $50 per year; but, as of June 2009, these laws have not yet been enacted, likely, I suspect, because of the pharmaceutical industry's intensive lobbying. States such as Pennsylvania and South Carolina employ "unsales" representatives to visit physicians and help them to prescribe medications based on the best scientific data instead of on the best sales pitches or the best physician/pharmaceutical rep relationships. The goal of these "unsales" reps is to save each respective state's Medicaid money on the out-of-control cost of medications. There are also objective, not-for-profit newsletters available to physicians, like the *Medical Letter* <www.medicalletter.org/>, where doctors can find information about medications without being influenced by pharmaceutical representatives.

Physicians can prescribe generic medications in place of brand-name medications. In fact, one of our local insurance companies, Excellus, has been giving physicians financial incentives (kickbacks?) to do so. The AMA states that accepting payment for switching medications could be an unethical violation of accepted practice.

Kickbacks aside, physicians who understand their biochemistry and pharmacology feel comfortable that there is bioequivalence, or similar effectiveness, between generic and brand-name meds. Thus they are willing to switch patients to less expensive prescriptions. But primary care physicians are more likely than specialists to prescribe generics. Primary care docs also tend to know better the difference in cost between brand-name and generic drugs.

Patients also prefer generics when possible to obtain them, due to the significant price difference between generics and non-generics. Even as a specialist, practically speaking, if the crunch came down to a patient either taking a generic or not taking any medication at all, certainly I would write for the generic.

Unfortunately, there are two names for every medication, the generic and the brand name. I used to kid my patients that medical school just was not hard enough, which was why they gave us two names to remember for each medication. (Thank God they did not test us on what the pills looked like!) That said, I was often concerned about switching patients' medications from the brand name to the generic, because of the high "mess up rate" in such changes. This problem was highlighted by one particular patient. She had requested changing all her many medications to generics, all at once. I was happy to oblige. I carefully wrote out for her, in my best handwriting, the names of the medications she was taking, why she was taking them, and then, next to each of the brand names, the name of the generic substitute. My goal for this patient and her husband, who accompanied her, was not to have any confusion as to what she would be taking. I thought that my little chart would eliminate that possibility. I was wrong. When she came back a couple of weeks later she was taking both the generic and the brand-name versions of some meds and had altogether stopped taking others. I learned my lesson. In the future I still was happy to switch patients to generics, but not all the meds at once.

Marketing Hides Behind Education

A portion of the pharmaceutical industry's marketing budget, whether they admit it or not, is for medical education. They sponsor and subsidize many of our national educational meetings to defray some of our costs. In return, they have additional marketing exposure. This is mostly legit. There are existing "pharma rules," put in place by our government in attempts to eliminate any improprieties between the pharmaceutical industry and physicians, although, as noted above, some think that these rules do not go far enough.

They need to be rigorously obeyed by both the physicians and the pharmaceutical companies, lest there be significant penalties dealt to individual pharmaceutical companies or even to physicians who speak on behalf of a pharmaceuticals.

Physicians are obligated to have about forty or fifty CME credits each year to keep us current with progress in medicine. Many of us fly to annual national meetings in distant, large, and expensive cities, to obtain these credits. Not only are significant costs involved in travel, food, and lodging, but there is also loss of income whenever we are not seeing patients, because this is the only way for most endocrinologists and primary care physicians to generate revenue.

Pharmaceutical companies help to organize the meetings by hiring independent medical education and communication companies to oversee arrangements, engage speakers, and choose topics. Yes, it is education for us, but it is also sales and marketing for the pharmaceutical companies. Marcia Angell reports on page 139 of her 2005 book that physicians prescribe more of the medications that are discussed at the meetings they attend.

At the actual meeting, the pharmaceutical companies set up elaborate marketing booths in the exhibit hall, which the doctors who helped to organize the meeting encourage us to visit. We are also wooed to the booths by the good-looking pharmaceutical representatives themselves, who offer us frozen yogurts, pretzels, and other *hazoray* in return for the opportunity to discuss and promote their drugs. I rationalized to myself that I needed to visit these booths, so that I could know what the other doctors were hearing and learning, and what was being told to my patients. I went along with the routine but, in my heart, it felt wrong.

"Thought Leader"? Who, Me?

What I am also not proud of, but also rationalize, was being a speaker on behalf of many pharmaceutical companies. As a speaker, I had the opportunity, several times each year, to go to speaker training meetings with hundreds of other physicians. I did not receive any CME credits at these meetings, because we were hired consultants and the meetings were considered promotional rather than educational. All the expenses to go to the meeting were paid by the pharmaceutical company that sponsored it, including round-trip air fare, food, and typically one night at a five-star hotel in some wonderful city like Orlando, Atlanta, or New York.

They also gave each of us a four-figure consultant's fee for attending the meeting and giving the company our opinions about their products. Some people call it an honorarium. Others, more crassly but maybe also more accurately, say the obvious, "They're buying us, *shtupping* us, to use and promote their drugs." I suspect that the companies had done their homework and that, for the money that they "paid" us, they got much more in return. In the end, the people who really paid for all this, once again, were the patients.

I rationalized that being a speaker helped me to learn, in intricate detail, about the pluses and minuses of the medications that I was prescribing to my patients anyway. I also gained opportunities to meet and to learn from other physicians in my field, which I relished, because, being too busy taking care of patients while in practice, I had little chance to discuss medical issues with other endocrinologists outside Syracuse. Going to speakers' meetings also credentialed me to deliver promotional programs when I returned home, on behalf of the sponsoring company, under very strict guidelines. In this connection, there was always a presentation by the company's in-house lawyers on the "do's and don'ts" of giving these promotional talks. This was where it got precarious.

The pharmaceutical companies believed that I, being a speaker or, as they called me, a "thought leader," would have influence over my peers in my community. When they first told me that I was a "thought leader," I kept looking over my shoulder like, "They can't be talking to me. They must be talking to the guy behind me."

The pharmaceutical company's *modus operandi* was obvious. If the other providers in our community heard from me, a "thought leader," and if they believed that I was honest, credible, and convinced that the medication was safe and effective to use, and that I used it, then maybe it would be OK for them to use it as well. That is multilevel marketing, and I am absolutely sure that it works. Otherwise, the pharmaceutical companies would not spend their time and certainly not large sums of money pursuing this sales approach. The kicker was that I would receive a four-figure "honorarium" — pay, money, dinero — from the sponsoring company for speaking at each program.

It took me many hours to prepare my presentations. So, the amount of money that I made per hour from speaking engagements was frequently about the same as from seeing patients in the office. One could use the analogy of how much a professional athlete makes for playing in one baseball game, or how much he earns per pitch, per catch, or per hit. What one does not see is how much time and effort the athlete, or me for that matter, put into preparing for the performance, behind the scenes, to be able to "play at that level."

These programs were usually at lunchtime in a physician's office or, if an evening event, at a nice restaurant — one that I could not easily afford to bring my family to on any regular basis — where I would receive a wonderfully prepared meal, including drinks, appetizers, and dessert. How could I sleep, knowing that I was doing something that might contribute toward maintaining the high costs of the very medications that I was prescribing to my own patients? Not easily, but here is my best shot. Rationalization is a much exalted defense mechanism.

First, I made quite clear to the representatives who invited me to speak at meetings that I would "tell" about, but would not "sell" or promote their drugs. Rather, I would discuss the pros and cons of their medications and include that information among several options to treat whatever disease process I may have been discussing.

Second, I felt like I was an ambassador for hypertension, hyperlipidemia, osteoporosis, thyroid disease, and diabetes awareness. Being able to speak at these meetings gave me opportunities to improve our understanding of these conditions and to help my peers diagnose and treat them. It was a service to my colleagues who, according to Daniel J. Rubin *et al.* in *Endocrine Practice*, January/February 2007, could use such help. This study concluded that, of the fifty-two internal medicine residents, twenty-one family practice residents, forty-two general surgery residents and forty-eight registered nurses who took a twenty-one-question survey regarding basic diabetes, the average score was only sixty-one per cent. A subgroup of the nurses had the highest score (eighty-two per cent). Primary care physicians take care of eighty-five per cent of all the diabetics in our country.

Third, as I was signed to speak for many competing companies, to promote one drug over another would have ruined my credibility and integrity. This was my own system of checks and balances. Above all, the one thing I want to take intact to my grave is my integrity. Much has been written about doctors pitching medications and thereby putting their integrity on the line. A paradigm case was when Pfizer pulled its Lipitor commercials in February 2008, under pressure from the U.S. House of Representatives Energy and Commerce Committee, whose probe had showed that they were misleading the public. Dr. Robert K. Jarvik had been a spokesperson for Lipitor and had contracted with Pfizer for two years at 1.35 million dollars to promote that drug. But Jarvik, the developer of the Jarvik-7 artificial heart, is a biomedical engineer, not a clinician. Even though he has an M.D. degree, he has always done just research, and has never been licensed to practice medicine.

The outcry from medical ethicists regarding physicians, or those impersonating medical practitioners, endorsing prescription medications or medical devices has been significant. In "Is Their Integrity on the Line When Doctors Pitch Products?" online at <www.ama-assn.org/amednews/>, Kevin B. O'Reilly cited Steven H. Miles, M.D., a prominent scholar of the Hippocratic Oath, and Howard Brody, M.D., Ph.D., a famous bioethicist, as each stating unequivocally that doctors should never endorse commercial products. Yet, on almost the other side of fence, O'Reilly cites an equally well known medical ethicist, Arthur L. Caplan, Ph.D., as saying that whether or not to help sell products is up to each doctor individually to decide. No one in the medical ethics field seems to be encouraging docs to pitch drugs or devices. All agree that conflict of interest exists in these cases. Would similar conflict of interest hold true for physicians who sell "nutritional supplements" out of their offices?

Fourth and last, I admit that significant time was required to prepare for the programs at which I spoke. I usually found this time on weekends or late at night, after all my patient work was done. Teaching required me to review old and learn new material, which helped to keep me sharp, better prepared to treat my own patients in the office. It also put variety into my day, rather than doing the same thing, day in and day out.

In "Dr. Drug Rep" in the November 25, 2007, Sunday *New York Times Magazine*, Daniel Carlat reported guesstimations that about twenty-five per cent of physicians are on pharmaceutical speaker training rosters or help to market pharmaceuticals in some other way. I suspect that more physicians would like to be involved, especially as insurance companies and Medicare lower their reimbursement rates for treating patients. Like everyone else, physicians are very interested in trying to, at least, maintain their incomes.

In medicine there is an unwritten rule called "Sutton's Law." Legend has it that Sutton's Law comes from a conversation with the notorious bank robber, Willie Sutton, who, when asked why he robbed banks, responded, "Because that's where the money is." We physicians invoke Sutton's Law when we try to diagnose a difficult medical case. We order first just the one test, like a biopsy, that will give us the best odds and the quickest chance of making a diagnosis. Some may also use Sutton's Law when describing the relationship between physicians and the pharmaceutical industry, because, for physicians, that *is* where the money is — perhaps to our patients' chagrin.

Despite my rationalizations, I still believe that my decision to collaborate with the pharmaceutical industry was wrong. It just did not feel good to be doing what I was doing. It was hard to put a finger on it, but in some respects my feel-

ing may have been analogous to U.S. Supreme Court Justice
Potter Stewart's definition of pornography: "I know it when I
see it." Anything that adds to patients' already gigantic costs,
which may subsequently adversely affect their health, I am
against. My litmus test for working with pharmaceutical companies was, "What would my patients say if they knew that I
was involved in these ventures?" I suspect that most of them
would feel disappointed, betrayed, even outraged. I am not
alone. Endocrinologists are typically among the medical specialists who receive the most money from drug companies.

The bottom line: As of June 2008, I have given my
last pharmaceutical-sponsored talk.

No WMDs Found in Iraq: Now I Do Not Know
What to Believe About Anything

Despite intelligence reports from the CIA, assurances from
President Bush, and statements by Colin Powell in front of the
whole world at the United Nations, there were no weapons of
mass destruction (WMDs) discovered in Iraq after the U.S. in-
vaded in 2003. Published medical studies contradict, supersede,
or overrule each other. Now I do not know what to believe
about anything. When patients or physicians asked me what I
thought about a particular study, especially one sponsored by
a pharmaceutical company, I frankly did not know what was
believable and what was not.

So what did I do? I tried to trust the FDA to be my
watchdog, to make sure that the new medications that came
out were safe. Unfortunately, their batting average has been
significantly less than 100 per cent. Many medications that
came to the market have subsequently been withdrawn:
Rezulin, Vioxx, Baychol, Zelnorm, Propulcid, etc., etc. etc.
Because of these medications, and others, that have been
removed from the market, I am never really certain anymore
about which drug is safe and which is not. Each time I prescribed a medication, I held my breath, not knowing whether
I would be helping or hurting this person.

There are two medications that I want to highlight to
make my point. First is hormone replacement therapy (HRT).

In the early 1990s it was thought that giving postmenopausal women HRT would not only improve their menopausal symptoms, like hot flashes, dysuria, and emotional lability, but also reduce their risks of having heart attacks or strokes. Because I was treating many women who had diabetes, hypertension, and hyperlipidemia, and thus were at high risk for these vascular conditions, I was urging them to start or stay on HRT. Then, out of the blue, in a 360-degree turn, the Heart and Estrogen/Progestin Replacement Study (HERS) came out, was reported in the August 19, 1998, *JAMA*, and suggested that HRT could actually *increase* the risk of heart attacks. The Women's Health Initiative (WHI) report in the July 17, 2002, *JAMA* essentially confirmed the HERS results. As Graham Chapman's King Arthur yelled to his knights when the French taunters lobbed a huge wooden rabbit at them in *Monty Python and the Holy Grail*, "RUN AWAY! RUN AWAY!" I then had to explain to all these women why my suggestion changed and I now wanted them off HRT, and worried they would never trust my suggestions or decisions again.

The second medication is Avandia. This diabetic medication was made available to the public in 1999. It was thought to be a safer version of a similar medication called Rezulin, which had been taken off the market a couple of years earlier, because of concerns about potentially fatal, drug-induced hepatitis. Avandia showed no evidence of causing hepatitis. In fact, there was evidence that it not only lowered blood sugars, but also, through a variety of different mechanisms, reduced the risk of heart attacks. It was touted as a way to treat diabetes and reduce the risk of vascular disease by several nationally renowned speakers and "thought leaders" in endocrinology, many of whom were also paid consulting fees by Glaxo Smith Kline (GSK), the manufacturer of Avandia. Their explanations were plausible and cogent. I bought into the concept. At my local programs, and to my patients, I offered Avandia as a medication that could improve glycemia as well as, theoretically, based upon its mechanism of action, reduce the danger from the number one killers of diabetics: heart attacks and strokes.

Then, on June 14, 2007, Dr. Steve Nissen, a prominent cardiologist from the Cleveland Clinic, and Kathy Wolski, M.P.H., published a meta-analysis in *NEJM*. Their study looked at forty-two different Avandia trials. It suggested that Avandia, like HRT, actually *increases* the risk of heart attacks and death. OUCH!!! Now what was any endocrinologist, or anyone else prescribing Avandia, to do? "RUN AWAY! RUN AWAY!"

As you may imagine, GSK refuted the claims and criticized the study. They had other prospective studies, that they had financed, that did not support the conclusions made in the meta-analysis. Therefore we needed a referee, like the FDA, to decide what the truth was. The FDA endocrine and diabetes subcommittee concluded, in a vote of 20-3, that Avandia did indeed increase the chance of heart attacks. Nevertheless, they also concluded, by a vote of 22-1, that it should not be taken off the market. This decision left many physicians in limbo for several months. What were we supposed to tell our patients?

I wonder how many of the members on that subcommittee were also "consultants" for GSK or their competitors.

The final FDA report, given on November 14, 2007, was to allow Avandia to stay on the market, but with explicit alerts that it should not be used in patients taking nitrates, such as nitroglycerin for people with angina, or insulin for diabetics. The FDA considered the conclusions of the Nissen/Wolski meta-analysis when it revised the existing black box warning that Avandia should not be used in people with advanced heart failure. But in the end, the FDA did not resolve whether Avandia increases or reduces the chance of heart attacks, or does neither. Should we clinicians stop using the medicine or continue prescribing it? Many physicians stopped prescribing Avandia, but some did not replace this drug with any other diabetic medication. Thus, through all the confusion, many diabetics' blood sugars increased, and so did their risks of diabetic complications.

I Did Not Really Know If I Was Helping Anyone

When I was in medical school and considering career options, I debated between internal medicine and surgery. I saw many bad outcomes from surgery and thought it might be too risky for my temperament. Being a doctor who would treat people with medications seemed less risky and I thought the hours would be better. I was zero for two, wrong on both counts. Not only were the hours comparable — we all work too much — but the medications can be as dangerous as surgery.

Frequently, drug reps would ask me how the medication that they were representing was working and whether I was seeing the same results as those described in their studies. I would usually respond, "I have no idea how this med is working or whether it's working at all." There are too many variables in taking care of real-life, non-study patients in clinical practice for a physician to be able to know how one medication may be influencing a patient's health. For example, did the blood sugars in this diabetic person improve because of the new medication, or because of reducing Mountain Dew consumption from twelve to six cans a day, or because of deciding to exercise, or because of eliminating a source of emotional stress, or because of a less painful lower back, or because ... ?

I never knew whether the treatment that I was giving people was doing any good. There is a statistic called "number needed to treat" (NNT). This means that I would have to treat a certain number of people with a particular medication before any one particular person would be likely to receive a benefit. For example, statins are a group of cholesterol-lowering medications that reduce the body's ability to manufacture cholesterol and thereby decrease the chance of having a heart attack or stroke. The NNT for a statin to prevent one heart attack or stroke is around thirty. Said another way, I would have to treat thirty people, who had each had either a heart attack or symptoms of heart disease, with a statin to reduce the chance of a heart attack or stroke in one person. The problem is that neither I nor anyone else ever knows who that one person is. Indeed, that person is not a real person, but only an abstract statistic. Thus I ended up treating more people with statins than necessary, risking many to potential side effects and saddling them with the cost of the medication.

Sometimes I would drive home from work at night wondering whether I was doing any good for anyone, other than the pharmaceutical company who was profiting mightily from my prescription. This was surely a hapless feeling.

I would like to believe that the medications that I have prescribed over the years have considerably reduced people's morbidity and rate of mortality. But I am not sure how many people I might have hurt along the way. My best suggestion for anyone who will listen is, "Don't get sick or hurt." That should reduce the chances of needing medications and of suffering their side effects.

We Need a Medication Derby

The pharmaceutical industry periodically develops new classes of medications to treat particular disease processes. Even in my relatively short career treating diabetes and other endocrinopathies, several new medications were developed that, I believe, helped my patients and were improvements over older medications. A good example is the newer insulins that have become available. A few years ago my son Sam said, "Dad, you are really bald and gray." "Sam," I said, "before I had you, I had a lot of hair and it was brown." In truth, it was not Sam that caused my hair changes; it was the older insulins, which had rather unreliable onset and duration of action. Patients had to eat all the time to prevent hypoglycemia (low blood sugar), because they never knew when the insulin was going to work. Still, not all "new" medications are really new. Many pharmaceutical companies rely on copycat medications, "me-too" drugs, to generate extra revenue and add to their profits.

"Me-too" drugs are meds that are manufactured by different pharmaceutical companies, but are not a new class of drugs. Rather, they are in many, if not most, ways the same as the meds produced by their original companies and already on the market. For example, there are two classes of blood pressure medications: angiotensin converting enzyme inhibitors (ACEIs) and angiotensin receptor blockers (ARBs). Each of these classes has over seven "me-too" drugs within it. There are six different statins. There are four similar osteoporosis medications that can be taken once a day, once a week, once a month, every three months, or even once a year. Do we need so many medications that all do virtually the same thing?

Clearly not. But they are easy for pharmaceutical companies to develop and pharmacologists know that they will work. When marketed correctly, these copycat drugs take some of the existing market shares from competitor companies and generate considerable returns on investments. In short, "me-too" drugs can be enormously profitable.

For physicians, "me-too" meds are really annoying. Let me explain. The drug reps are able, through outside agencies, to monitor and track physicians' prescribing habits, a process called "prescription data mining," in which, as Carlat described it on page 68, "specialized pharmacy-information companies ... buy prescription data from local pharmacies, repackage it, then sell it to pharmaceutical companies." The AMA is also indirectly involved, by releasing physician numbers from the federal Drug Enforcement Administration (DEA), which then allows these prescription mining companies to match DEA numbers with physicians' names. The AMA makes millions of dollars in this way. I feel that the whole process is an invasion of my privacy.

If one of the "me-too" reps found out that I was prescribing more of their competitor's drug, they would detail me even harder by giving me the full court press and increasing their doses of friendship. They would also make more trips to my office, give me more samples, bring more treats (*chatchkas* and *hazoray*) and free lunches for my staff, and even stalk me in the hospital. They would find out my patient rounding routine and then just happen to be in the lobby of the hospital when I walked through. They would offer me the opportunity to speak on behalf of their company and turn up the adulation meter, "Dr. Lebowitz, you are a thought leader. Everyone in Syracuse wants to know what you think." Yeah, right!

One way to solve the "me-too" drug problem would be to hold a contest among the makers of the respective "me-too" drugs, a veritable "medicine derby." Studies would be designed and run by independent officials who would have absolutely no financial ties to, or any other conflict of interest with, any of the contestants. The prize would be winner-take-all. That way I would know, if my patients needed medications from that class of drugs, that they would be receiving the best on the market, not just what was best promoted or advertised. The price of the winning medication should not then increase, even though there would be no further competition, because the winning company's expenses for marketing it should go down. They may then even be able to charge our patients less and still make the same profit, as their cost of doing business declines.

In the future, if another company wanted to challenge the existing medication in the same class, like a contender wanting to take on the boxing champ, the challenger would have to show that its new drug worked better than the existing drug, not just better than placebo or a sugar pill. Then the FDA would approve the new drug and decertify the existing one.

Having such derbies would also reduce the time and energy spent by the physicians and mid-level providers who try to be fair to all the companies producing "me-too" drugs by trying to prescribe them all equally. I have had conversations with pharmaceutical reps telling them that I was trying to prescribe all the medications in the same class equally. One retorted, "I looked at the stat sheet and saw that you prescribed my competitor's drug twenty-five per cent more than mine ..." I suggested that he not come back to my office ever again. Then there was one less "me-too" drug to prescribe.

Chapter Fifteen

What I Will Not Miss About Treating Patients

Adherence — Lifestyle

Before the 2006 Super Bowl a patient of mine, with obesity, diabetes, sleep apnea, and elevated blood pressure and cholesterol, told me he looked forward to going to a Super Bowl party because it was an "opportunity" to eat. He did not know who was going to be playing nor did he really care. He was going for the food. What my patient failed to realize was that his body did not care if it was the Super Bowl, Christmas, New Year's, or Tuesday. If he ate more calories than he needed he would gain weight and his already fragile medical problems would get worse. There were no free days when his body would say, "Go ahead and eat as much as you want of whatever you like, this day is on me. Those calories don't count and you won't gain weight." I will not miss such episodes of dietary indiscretion and the associated deterioration of my patients' medical conditions.

If I ever run for political office, my platform would be: "Get rid of the month of December." December was when many of my patients with diabetes and metabolic problems got worse. There were leftovers from Thanksgiving, numerous holiday parties, the usual array of birthdays and anniversaries, not to mention Christmas Eve, Christmas day, Hanukkah, and New Year's Eve celebrations. Did I mention Kwanzaa?

The average American, based on self-reporting studies, was thought to gain between five and ten pounds during the winter holidays, but "A Prospective Study of Holiday Weight Gain" in the March 23, 2000, *NEJM* suggested only about a one-pound gain. Everyone knows that putting weight on is easy, but taking it off is the challenge. The number one New Year's resolution is to go on a diet; but, as everyone also knows, the success rate for achieving any of our New Year's resolutions is not very good.

What was most frustrating to me, the one who was

desperately trying to help patients whose corpulence was negatively impacting many of their other medical problems, was that I could not beat their overeating habits. If there were a war between the medications that I prescribed and the patients' eating behaviors, their behaviors would always win, and as a consequence their health would lose. This does not mean I was not empathetic with their situations. After all, I am human too and have similar weaknesses for good-tasting food. However, I did not always accept their dietary noncompliance, especially because they all knew better. They were repeatedly educated by me, my staff, my dietician, and my diabetic educator regarding the negative consequences of overeating. Evidently, emotions trump intellect when it comes to eating behaviors.

I had to be tactful. Terms like "obesity," "fatness," "large size," "big-boned," or "excess fat" can be undesirable or even offensive to people who weighed more than they wanted or should. Using any of them might make my efforts counterproductive.

People whose weight was heavier than they wanted it to be were frequently referred to me to determine whether their weight problems were "glandular," due to their "metabolism," or from some other cause. Frankly, I am not sure why I am certified in diabetes, endocrinology, *and* metabolism, as I cannot easily measure metabolism, nor are there any medications to change metabolism. The best way to improve one's metabolism is to exercise, which increases muscle mass. Muscle burns more calories at rest than the same amount of fat. Nonetheless, the referred patients would pray that they had adrenal problems, pituitary maladies, or thyroid conditions. They insisted that, even though their tests were in the normal range, these results were not "normal" for them. Sometimes, to help them work through the issues, and once and for all to determine whether their weight was due to thyroid hormone deficiency or not, I would give them a trial of some thyroid hormone. To their chagrin, especially if they did not change their eating or exercise routines, their weight would not change.

Yogi Berra is supposed to have said, among many other sayings, "Baseball is ninety per cent mental. The other half is physical." The same is true for people's eating behavior.

Thus, "Half the battle of losing weight is ninety per cent mental." I have treated countless people with weight-related health problems, and know that their weight is affected not only by their genetic predispositions to gain weight (the so-called "thrifty gene") and by what and how much they eat, but also by their emotions, i.e., by how and why they eat.

People will eat or overeat because they are sad or happy, celebrating or mourning, bored or frustrated, stressed or relaxed. I knew that I could not control my patients' glycemia, blood pressure, lipids, sleep apnea, arthritis, or depression until I had first helped them to gain control over their own eating habits. If I asked my overweight patients what would be the one thing that they would change about themselves if they could, they would almost always say their weight. I know that they did not want to have issues with their weight, but frequently the problem became a vicious circle. The more they ate, the more unhappy they became, and the more unhappy they became, the more they ate.

Because, for many of my patients, their weight was the root of their medical conditions and, for most of these, their eating behaviors were the root of their weight problems, I tried to help them with these behaviors by discussing the issues openly, compassionately, and honestly with them in the office. I reinforced to them that they did not need to look waiflike and that even small amounts of weight loss, like five per cent of their total body weight, could have salutary effects. I gave them handouts with strategies on how not to "stress eat" and about how even small amounts of excess calories over long periods of time can lead to substantial weight gain. I sent them to dieticians and diabetic educators to help them understand the impacts of their food choices. I referred them to psychologists who specialized in eating disorders, even though insurance companies frequently would not approve these referrals. I even prescribed anorectics, antidepressants, or anxiety medications to try to curb their behaviors, hoping to limit their use of prescribed medications to treat the complications of their weight, such as diabetes, hypertension, and hyperlipidemia. I became a behaviorist or *de facto* psychiatrist in addition to being a diabetologist. As a last resort, I sent some of my patients for weight loss surgery. Even with its inherent risks, bariatric surgery is the best treatment option in 2009 to achieve the most significant and sustainable weight loss over the longest period of time.

There were times when I saw my patients getting breakfast in the cafeteria and witnessed first-hand what food choices some of them made: two donuts or muffins and a can of soda, for example. It was even more uncomfortable if they saw me when they were out to dinner, especially if they were eating delectable desserts. Sometimes I wished that I had a one-way mirror to see what their behaviors were at home, particularly the people who insisted that they "don't eat anything." I certainly did not want to judge them. I am not perfect with my food choices either, nor do I enjoy being judged, but I certainly wanted to understand them, with the goal of helping them. I also admit that sometimes, out of absolute frustration, I wanted to say, "What the hell are you doing?" I was incensed that they were sabotaging their own health, which I was spending enormous amounts of time and energy desperately trying to salvage.

To maintain or lose weight, you need to burn more calories than you take in. This is a simple application of the first law of thermodynamics, i.e., energy is always conserved, either being stored in some form or used and thereby converted into some other form. Therefore, exercise is a key component in controlling weight. The first question that I always asked my patients with weight problems was, "Do you like to exercise?" If the answer was no, then my success rate at motivating or encouraging them to do something that they did not enjoy doing, like exercising, was low, especially when it competed with all the other things in life that they needed to do. As alternatives, I would suggest counting each day's steps with an inexpensive pedometer and burning more calories in daily activities by, for example, walking stairs instead of using elevators, getting up to change TV channels instead of using remote controls, or parking farther away from store entrances.

Usually people who do not like to exercise have several excuses, like, "It's too hot in the summer and too cold in the winter." I kidded with them that, here in Central New York, there might be three good days each year when the weather is just right to exercise.

It was also demoralizing to me, and probably to patients as well, to watch their weight go back up and their medical conditions exacerbate, especially after they had lost weight by dieting and exercising. I called these my "Mae West" patients; "When they were good, they were very good, but when they were bad, they were very bad."

By the way, although some physicians are proud to exclaim that *they* were able to get their patients to lose weight, I personally do not believe that I was able to get my patients to do anything that they did not want to do, no matter how enthusiastically or persuasively I may have encouraged them.

People frequently want to know what their ideal weight should be. The practical answer, according to me, Dr. Mick, and not the life insurance tables, is "a weight that keeps you looking good and feeling well, while limiting or eliminating medical conditions that could be associated with weighing too much." We need new ideas to help our citizens achieve their "ideal body weight," lest our health care system go "belly up."

It is clear that our health providers' attempts to modify our population's behavior are not working, whether regarding diets, education, or medication. A cardiovascular endocrinologist in Virginia, Dr. Joseph Chemplavil, advocated "Dieting For Dollars" to encourage his patients to lose weight. He would give them one dollar for each pound they lost between office visits. Conversely, they would give him one dollar for each pound they gained. His idea is intriguing. I think that money is a powerful motivator. After all, why do we stop at stop signs and try not to speed on our roadways? Because, if we get caught, it can cost us a lot of money. OK, speeding is dangerous too, but so is being heavyset.

Although it may sound draconian, maybe there should be a "weight tax":

If you wanted to purchase calorie-dense foods like those from fast food restaurants, and if your BMI were in the overweight or obese range, you would have to pay a surcharge, much like the extra taxes on cigarettes. New York State raised its cigarette excise tax again, on June 3, 2008, another $1.25, making the total state tax $2.75 per pack. Antismoking advocates expected that this extra cost would induce more than 100,000 people to quit smoking, thus reducing the medical consequences and costs associated with cigarettes. Would a "weight tax" achieve the similar goals of people eating better, eating less, and subsequently suffering fewer medical problems and reducing their health care costs?

Health care costs could be dramatically reduced if something as "simple" as our citizens' behaviors could change and if preventable medical conditions, like diabetes, hypertension, and hyperlipidemia, could be avoided or delayed. Employers have a stake in the game. Studies that correlate medical claims data with individual risk factors show that corpulent, physically inactive employees with diabetes are more likely to get sick and as a consequence increase health care costs.

Social issues also need to be considered when discussing and evaluating the obesity epidemic. Food, desserts, and the proliferation of calorie-dense, inexpensive fast food in restaurants all add to the problem. Lisa Graham reported in the January 1, 2006, issue of *American Family Physician* on the Rand Corporation study released on October 5, 2005, which had suggested that weight gain in children may be associated with the cost of fresh produce. For example, children in Mobile, Alabama, where produce costs were the highest of the fifty-nine urban areas studied, gained fifty per cent more weight than the national average. Clearly, a multipronged approach to new medical and social policies is necessary to curb our country's "ever bulging" weight.

Adherence — Medications

Years ago in my waiting room I put a sign the size of California that read, "BRING YOUR MEDICATION LIST OR YOUR PILL BOTTLES TO EVERY OFFICE VISIT." The request seemed pretty straightforward and uncomplicated to me. Many patients followed my request beautifully. Others were not as reliable. So, when they came in without either their med lists or their pill bottles, I asked them if they had seen the sign in the waiting room. The most common response: "What sign?" The conversation went on. "Don't worry doc, I know all my pills. I take a small blue one, a round red one, a funny shaped white one ..." UUGGHH!!!

The large sign certainly was not to harass my patients, but to reduce the chance of medication errors. According to NIH data from July 2006, medication errors harm 1.5 million people and kill several thousand each year costing the nation 3.5 billion dollars annually. An October 2006 study from the Feinberg School of Medicine at Northwestern University showed that forty per cent of 119 surveyed patients could not remember what medications they were on. That percentage was sixty among patients with "low health literacy," i.e., those who had difficulty reading relatively simple medical literature or understanding health-related issues.

One of my mentors used to say, "If you know the patient's medications, then you'll know what medical conditions the patient has." But what if the patient did not know the medications? Many times the patient would retort, "You're my doctor. You should know what medications I'm on." Or, many of the men would say, "I take whatever my wife gives me." They are so trusting. Did they never hear of the Black Widow? Some would say, "I'm still on the same ones as last time," but, when the list was read to them, there were almost always changes. Many of my patients were seen by several different providers, who each prescribed medications, and I was not always notified of these changes.

A study released by Medco Health Solutions in September 2006 concluded, after reviewing drug insurance claims from 2.4 million adults in 2004, that senior citizens were at the greatest risk of prescription or medication errors, and that this error rate increased proportionately to the number of doctors and the number of drugs per patient. For example, seniors who were treated by two doctors received an average of twenty-seven prescriptions each year and risked ten errors, but those with five doctors averaged forty-two prescriptions and risked sixteen errors.

FPA spent considerable amounts of money instituting an EMR system. It was supposed to reduce the chance of errors, especially by pharmacists trying to read our handwriting, and equally as important, to make us more efficient, so that we could see even more patients in the same amount of time, without having to write prescriptions by hand. Many physicians who use EMR swear by it, although the rate of its usage by all providers has been slowed, not only by the prohibitive start-up costs of purchasing all its hardware, but also by the learning curve to become familiar with the system. Concurrent is a loss of revenue associated with seeing fewer patients early on.

What is also limiting about EMR is that there are many different systems available from many different companies and they cannot communicate with each other. For example, if a patient had a new prescription given by a physician just seen, or had a laboratory or x-ray study done during an ER visit, then showed up in my office the next day, I could not access the new prescription, labs, or any tests or reports. My nurses would still have to get on the phone and call the appropriate doctor or hospital, navigate to the person who might be able to help with answers, and, if they had time on the other end, to fax over the information while the patient was still in my office.

Would it not be ideal if all the systems could communicate with each other, or if each patient had a CD, a "smart card" as is common in Taiwan, or even an implanted computer chip, which could be updated at each encounter with a provider and which the next provider could download? Think how much unnecessary testing could be eliminated if each provider had instant access to each patient's data bank.

Some patients have not caught up with this notion. They believe that all these computers can talk with each other. They also believe that the computers are completely accurate, not understanding the concept of "junk in equals junk out." In our system, we had all the patients' medications listed, although at certain times there were errors, especially if the patients had given us the wrong information or if the nurse who had entered the data had been rushed or distracted. The system was actually far from infallible. I am still not convinced that using computers could limit medical errors any better than a careful clinician or nurse taking more time with patients, or the patients reliably bringing in their medication lists or all their medication bottles. Despite all these problems, some patients, particularly those taking many medications, would typically say, "Look on your computer, that's my list."

Although pill boxes and medication lists do help, I admit that it was difficult for many of my patients who were taking polypharmacy, i.e., a multitude of different medications, to remember what pills they were taking, why they were taking these pills, and even just to take them. There have been times when I myself had to take a pill for a finite period of time, yet had a hard time remembering to take it each day, even with my symptoms to remind me.

I understand why some patients miss taking their meds. Many of the conditions I treated, like type 2 diabetes, hypertension, hyperlipidemia, and osteoporosis, are asymptomatic. Studies have shown that adherence to medications is worst for people with medical conditions that do not have obvious symptoms. It makes intuitive sense that adherence to medications is much better for people who have symptoms, like back pain or heartburn. They take their meds and their symptoms go away, at least temporarily.

Nonetheless, it was frustrating for me to have spent time listening to a patient's history, doing examinations, ordering the correct blood and imaging tests, making a diagnosis, explaining the diagnosis, and then prescribing a medication, only to have the patient not adhere to the therapy and thus not have the condition improve. (I am not here talking about patients who do not take their medications because of high costs or side effects.) Why do non-adherent patients waste everyone's time, energy, and money? The Japanese have the highest costs for medications in the world, but their noncompliance rate is only three per cent, contrasted to our rate of twenty-nine per cent, according to *Medical News Today* <www.medicalnewstoday.com/articles/93397.php> of January 9, 2008.

What was even more disturbing to me was when people said they were taking their medicine and then, through lab testing, we found out that they were not. That was always an uncomfortable phone conversation: "Hello Mr. Jones, this is Dr. Lebowitz. Your cholesterol level is very high. It does not appear that the current medication is working for you. I need to change your medication. What's that? You haven't been taking the medicine? But when you came to the office you said you were taking it ..." What was worse, because it was dangerous, was when patients' blood tests were abnormal and they swore that they were taking a medication like thyroid pills or insulin. I then would increase the dose of that medication. If they then started taking it adherently, at the higher doses, it could kill them. Patient deaths were something that I usually tried to avoid.

I admit that some people became very religious about taking their medications, and sometimes also about adjusting their lifestyles, after near life-ending events like heart attack or stroke. Others did not need such near-death experiences to encourage them to take their medicines. One of my colleagues coined the term, "DDW." It means "dick don't work," a less politically correct way of saying "erectile dysfunction." He believed that many of his male diabetics became more adherent with their diabetes medications when they started suffering from DDW.

I believe that I understand human nature "somewhat." After all, I sat in my exam rooms day after day and year after year listening to people's stories and observing their behaviors. It remains an enigma to me why some people would not do many of the things necessary to prevent problems, whether lifestyle changes or taking their medications. Instead they dared a medical problem to attack them, assuming the "It won't happen to me" posture, even when they knew very well that it could.

End of Life

Many years ago, I admitted an elderly woman, whom I had never met before, to the hospital after she suffered a massive, near fatal heart attack. In the ER she had malignant arrhythmias requiring repeated shocks to her heart. She survived, but was left with an extraordinarily weak heart muscle, which resulted in congestive heart failure, respiratory failure necessitating being on a ventilator, and coma from hypoxic brain injury. She stayed in the cardiac care unit (CCU) for weeks, suffering one complication after another, including repeated bouts of pneumonia, urinary tract infections, liver and kidney dysfunction, and gastrointestinal bleeding, to name a few. We performed a tracheostomy, endoscopy, and placed a feeding tube into her stomach, central lines into her large veins, and catheters into her arteries and bladder. Despite our "working out on her," we all knew that her prognosis was nil. Her son stayed in her room day and night, monitored staff activity, kept written notes of all staff interactions, and refused to "let her go." "First, do no harm." But each day, and sometimes twice a day, I walked into her room and thought, "What am I doing?" I am not helping this poor woman. Rather, I thought, I was torturing her. As the days and weeks went on with no progress and only setbacks, I was becoming demoralized. Then one day, miraculously, she opened her eyes. She wanted to try to speak. We adjusted her tracheostomy so that she could talk. She blurted three words in a hoarse, guttural tone: "LET ... ME ... DIE!" Then she closed her eyes and never spoke again.

Despite those words, her son refused to let nature take its course. He implored the staff to persist with her care. Even though I had treated countless sick patients in ICUs, I became so despondent treating this poor woman, especially after she had uttered those three words, that I asked the chief of the CCU to take over for me. Subsequently, there were frequent meetings with all the staff and her son. Even our hospital administrators and ethics committee members met with him, but he remained steadfast that he wanted everything done, at all costs — as long as Medicare and the insurance company were paying for it. He threatened lawsuit if not. Several more months went by before she eventually passed away. She never woke up again and remained on a ventilator until the very end.

I had another case, a sixtyish-year-old man with terminal Lou Gehrig's disease, amyotrophic lateral sclerosis. I became his primary care physician by default, because he had steroid-induced diabetes associated with his liver transplant. As his respiratory muscles gradually weakened from his underlying disease, he was hospitalized multiple times for pneumonia and eventually required full ventilator support. His mentation deteriorated and he gradually slipped into a coma. There were many opportunities for him to go naturally. However, his family, who were incredibly kind, caring, and loving, could not bear to see him go. At his family's insistence, he spent his last year at home, on a ventilator and comatose, with all paid for by the government and his insurance policy.

During that last year of his life, I was on the phone with his family or his visiting nurses several times a week, "working out on the patient," adjusting his tube feedings, insulin, and steroid doses, as well as treating recurrent urinary tract infections, pneumonias, and bedsores. Although I admired the family for their commitment to their beloved, it all just seemed wrong. I cared deeply for the patient too, but was relieved when he succumbed to his illness.

Although these two cases may seem like extremes, in many ways they are representative of end-of-life care in the U.S. and will likely become even more common as the baby boomers age and develop chronic diseases. The chance of dying goes up with the number of chronic diseases. During the final year of life, Medicare beneficiaries average about four major or chronic illnesses.

Although most patients say they wish to die at home, as their ancestors did before 1900, when just about everyone died at home, most Medicare patients spend at least some time in the hospital during their last year of life and far too many die either in the hospital or in a nursing home. This prompts asking, what about the costs to treat people during the last year of their life?

We all must remember that no matter how much treatment we, as physicians, administer to people, eventually everyone will die. I felt like I did nothing to improve the quality of life of these two patients and many others, and, although I followed the AMA guidelines on end-of-life care, I felt like I may have caused them additional pain and suffering, a thought I try to suppress as quickly as it enters my mind.

Trust: The Backbone of All Relationships

Mr. T. had type 1, insulin-dependent diabetes, but also had enormous muscles like Samson, Hercules, the Hulk, or the real "Mr. T.," but without the Mohawk hairdo and all the bling. He complained of intermittent loss of libido and erectile dysfunction. When I measured his level of testosterone, the male hormone, it was low. I always considered that being a physician was like being a glorified riddle-solver. The riddle in this case was, "What can make a man look like he was taking anabolic steroids, even if he denied it, yet have decreased libido, ED, and a low testosterone level?" Frankly, the most likely answer, despite his insistence that he was not "juicing," was that he was taking anabolic or androgenic steroids. What was I to do?

Without accusing him, I discussed with him the potential negative consequences of taking steroids, including infertility, development of breast tissue, and emotional lability, in addition to the pitfalls of taking over-the-counter "nutritional supplements." I gave him Viagra to help with his intermittent ED and frequently checked his testosterone levels over the ensuing years. Sometimes his testosterone was normal and other times it was low, another signal that he was intermittently "doping."

Also, despite his insistence that he was taking his insulin according to instructions, his hemoglobin A1c, a measure of the blood sugar average over the previous two to three months, was also considerably elevated. This was another indication of him not being forthright with me.

I liked Mr. T., but I just could not believe him enough to feel that I was really doing a good job medically for him. I was suspicious of everything he told me. Clearly, the backbone of all solid relationships, whether personal or professional, is trust. I was best able to serve my patients when I knew that they were honest in discussing their issues with me. Mr. T. was not unique.

Another florid example of a patient not being forthright was when a thirty-something-year-old woman, who worked as an emergency medical technician (EMT) on an ambulance, was having recurrent syncopal episodes, passing out spells, which, interestingly, only occurred when she was at work. During her faints, she was noted to have hypoglycemia. Eventually, she was brought to the ER during a spell and I was summoned to evaluate her. I measured her insulin levels and gave her other tests to help me discover whether her low blood sugar was due to her body making too much insulin, a condition called an insulinoma, or if she was surreptitiously taking insulin or other diabetes medications to lower her blood sugar intentionally. Why would anyone do such a thing as taking insulin to lower one's own blood sugar down from healthy levels? As it turned out, her boyfriend worked on the same ambulance with her, but evidently he was not paying enough attention to her. If she could attract more notice from him, that would be what doctors call "secondary gain" from her condition.

Some women may be direct and say something to their boyfriends, while others may try to beautify themselves, and yet others may look for new boyfriends. But this particular woman had decided to get his attention by taking insulin to induce hypoglycemia. How do I know for sure that she took insulin, despite her fervently denying it, even when she was caught with her hand in the "cookie jar"? Her blood tests were 99.9 per cent reliable, but I did not confront her until I had gone through a lot of medical literature describing case reports of other people who had intentionally induced hypoglycemia. With the help of one of my professors, I came up with a new calculation, to make sure that our labs had been 100 per cent accurate in determining that my patient had indeed taken insulin. We published this innovation in the March 8, 1993, issue of *Archives of Internal Medicine.* Her intense denial was not unique. Case reports described other people who had denied taking insulin surreptitiously, even until their death. Confronting my patient, including telling her the risks of taking insulin, was one of the least pleasurable, yet most memorable, conversations that I have ever had with anyone. I never heard from her again.

I'm Your Pusher Man

I met C.N., then in her thirties, during my first days in fellowship, 1989. She had been referred to our diabetes clinic by her primary care physician to help control her type 1 diabetes, which had been diagnosed only a few months earlier. Her primary care doc had first assumed that, because she was older, her disease was type 2 diabetes, and had started her on ineffective oral diabetic medications. The medical literature well describes that about half of the people with type 1 diabetes are diagnosed after the age of twenty, hence the change in terminology in the late twentieth century from "juvenile onset diabetes" or "juvenile diabetes" to "type 1 diabetes." Such patients need insulin to control their blood sugars, which is what

I prescribed for her. Soon thereafter her blood sugars improved and all her hyperglycemic signs and symptoms resolved.

Yet she developed lower extremity edema, an unusual, very uncomfortable, albeit short-lived consequence of insulin therapy. I prescribed diuretics to palliate the condition, but, even after the edema abated, she complained of persistent discomfort in her legs. There were no objective findings, such as skin lesions, inflammation of her joints, varicosities of her veins, diminished pulses, delayed capillary refill, or neurological signs. I treated her conservatively with Motrin-like medications and Tylenol, but over time her pains persisted and intensified.

I then ordered a variety of imaging studies to assess her venous and arterial blood supply, her bones and joints, and her neurological system, but all the tests came back negative. Because her pains were increasing, I had to use stronger analgesics to keep her comfortable. Eventually I gave her narcotics.

C.N. was understandably becoming more frustrated with the lack of diagnosis and the continued pain. Her husband, who accompanied her to all her office visits, was equally distressed. She could not do anything except lie on the couch all day, too tired and uncomfortable for anything else.

I referred her to a neurologist, a rheumatologist, a vascular surgeon, a psychiatrist, and a pain management specialist. No one could find any objective reason for her pains but the psychiatrist did not believe that her symptoms were psychosomatic. What was I left to do except continue to prescribe narcotics, which she took religiously every six hours? Month after month, year after year, I would get phone calls from C.N. asking me to refill her narcs, as I was only willing to give her one month's supply at a time. I dreaded those phone calls. They reminded me that I did not know why she was in constant pain, that she was likely addicted to the opioids, and that I was her "pusher man."

When My Best Just Was Not Good Enough

P.C., an upbeat, youthful looking person with a good attitude, was also referred to my office by her primary care physician to help manage her brittle type 1 diabetes. She had been diagnosed with this condition about forty years prior when she was about five years old. She already had seen several different diabetes specialists in our community, all without benefit. Her blood sugars were like "The Hulk" roller coaster at Universal Studios, up and down and all around many times without rhyme or reason. The worst part was that, after over forty years of diabetes, despite having had no diabetic micro- or macrovascular complications of her diabetes, she had lost her ability to sense hypoglycemia. The ability to feel your blood sugars when they are low can be lifesaving for anyone, especially someone with diabetes.

The first thing P.C. told me when she came to my office for her initial visit was, "I know your reputation and I know you will help me. If you can't, no one can. I am not ready to die. I want to live."

For years my diabetic educator and I worked diligently trying to help P.C. We tweaked her insulins, trying different types, and changed her doses according to whether she was active or not. We changed the times she took her insulins and the places where she injected them into her body. We tried different diets, taught her carbohydrate counting, all along ruling out other medical conditions that could have affected her blood sugar control, like thyroid disease, adrenal disease, or gastroparesis. We spoke with her by phone at least a couple of times each week, trying to stabilize her blood sugar level at somewhere between 150 and 400 milligrams per deciliter before meals. (Normal blood sugars for people without diabetes are between 70 and 100 mg/dL before meals.)

Despite all these efforts by the patient, my staff, and me, her blood sugars fluctuated like the Dow Jones industrial average at the end of 2008. Worst of all, she continued to have episodes of hypoglycemia without awareness. I lost track of how many times I received phone calls from her family or boyfriend(s) notifying me that they had found her unconscious and needed to either inject her with the antidote for her hypoglycemia, glucagon, or call 911.

Finally, after years of resisting being put on an insulin pump, afraid that the pump would malfunction and leave her worse than she already was, she agreed to go on it. The insulin pump is not an artificial pancreas, and certainly not a panacea, but provides insulin in reliable and flexible doses. We hoped that it would give her the best chance of maintaining reasonable blood sugars, without her typically extreme highs and lows.

P.C. spent considerable time with me and my diabetic educator, learning the intricacies of the pump to the point where she was an expert. We spoke with her by phone every day for the first two weeks that she was on the pump and saw her in the office a few times, to make sure that all was going as well as possible, given her initial reluctance to go on the pump. Then it happened. I got the phone call that I never wanted to get. It was from the coroner. P.C., who lived alone and was very independent, had been found dead in her bed that morning by her family. I broke down and cried. Of all the people to fail, I did not want it ever to be P.C. She was always upbeat and positive, willing to give maximal effort to deal with her diabetes curse. All she wanted from me was help to treat her condition and I had let her down. My best was just not good enough.

I needed an explanation for her death. Her family agreed to an autopsy. It showed that all her organs were fine, despite forty years of diabetes. There was no evidence of any diabetic complications! Who knows how long she could have lived if not for the ultimate cause of her death: "hypoglycemia."

The family also gave us her insulin pump and glucometer to investigate, to see if she had had any missteps with managing her blood sugars. The pump was working fine and her blood sugar level before she went to bed the night she died was about 400. Because of that, she had done exactly what she had been instructed to do, i.e., take just one measly unit of insulin to bring her blood sugars as gently as possible down into a more reasonable range. She felt lousy whenever her blood sugars were too high. That one unit did her in.

I went to her wake a couple of days after her death. I talked with her family and gave my condolences. I then stood by her casket, looked her in the eye, apologized to her for letting her down, and told her I would miss her dearly.

Can't Please Them All

Ms. P. was a twenty-year-old woman, wheelchair bound, and only minimally communicative due to the consequences of a brain tumor that she had had several years prior. She was referred to me by my friend, a family practitioner, who was concerned that she had a hormonal problem, because she was gaining weight rapidly, was not having her periods, and was developing hirsutism (unwanted hair growth) on her face. My heart broke for this young woman. Her life, as she knew it, was forever changed by that tumor. Over many months and several office visits I worked diligently with her and her mother, who always accompanied her to my office, trying to make her diagnosis, instituting her treatment plan, and then following her up to see if the treatment was working. In short, I wanted to do anything I could to try to make her days better — which was my motto for all the patients I treated.

Then, unfortunately, at what ended up being our last office visit, I was unusually delayed in seeing her at the scheduled time. This was not because I had taken an extra long lunch break, nor had I double booked, nor had I been sitting in my office with my feet on the desk reading the *Sports Illustrated* swimsuit issue before having a nap. There had been urgencies that I had needed to deal with, as well as unexpected issues that I had needed to address for other scheduled patients before I saw her. Those kinds of days, which felt like they would never end and happened more times than I care to remember, were the most stressful of all. I was desperate to keep up with the intense patient demands in my allotted time, all while trying to keep my composure, even though I felt like I could lose it at any moment.

As was my custom, out of courtesy to the patient, especially since I am impatient at waiting myself, if I knew that I was going to be delayed more than thirty minutes to see a patient, I would have someone on my staff go to the waiting room, notify the patient of the delay, and give the patient the option of either waiting longer or rescheduling for another time. This is exactly what was done for my twenty-something patient and her mother. Most people are mindful that I am just one person trying to serve the needs of many. However, even though I came into the exam room profusely apologizing for keeping them waiting so long, her mother laid into me for being inconsiderate and uncaring. Inconsiderate and uncaring?! I felt like all I did every day was give until I had nothing left in the tank, and then I would search for some more to give. Though, initially, I was sorry for their inconvenience, I admit that I lost my patience and told them to leave the office when the mother would not let up. All people, even nice guys, have their breaking points. What did I think about while I was driving home that day and when I was trying to fall asleep that night? Not the many people that I helped, but the one person who rang my bell. Sometimes, trying to live by the adage of not going to sleep mad at anyone, I would even call the disgruntled patients at home at night, trying to make amends.

Also, it always disappointed me when a patient came into my office and was critical of the kindness and compassion of one of my doctor friends, physicians whom I know to be the "nicest of the nice." Patients did not appreciate that when they saw one of these doctors, in that snapshot of time, the doctor may have been under significant pressure, trying to manage many complicated patient problems, or behind in the schedule, or exhausted from the pace of the day, or experiencing problems at home. Doctors whom patients only meet once may not always be at their "friendliest best." All physicians are vulnerable to the same.

No Shows

Each weekend I would review numerous patient charts, trying to resolve complicated problems that I did not have time or energy for during the weekdays or nights. This meant taking time away from my family or from activities that I wanted to do for myself, including just unwinding and recuperating enough to be able to play at my peak the following week. My ultimate goal was to be able to walk into my office at 7:30 a.m. Monday ready to see my first patient, with all the loose ends from the week before tied up, all outstanding issues resolved, and the score tied at 0-0.

Then it would happen! The first two patients that Monday morning would not show up! No shows!

Sometimes I prayed for no shows, like when I was running miserably late seeing patients, feeling tightness in my chest and neck like a wrestler's choke hold, or like when I did not have enough time to think through anyone's problems and just wished that the next person I saw would only say, "I'm fine, Doc, I just need my prescription filled and I can be on my way."

But most other times I resented the no shows. It tried my patience when patients did not come in first thing Monday morning as expected, especially as we had called everyone the business day before. All I could think about at such times, as I mulled around the office and made small talk with my staff, was, "Why did I waste my free time this weekend reviewing those charts, time I could have used so many other ways, when I could have done them this morning? If I had only known that the Monday morning patients weren't going to come!"

I always appreciated patients who called at least twenty-four hours in advance of their appointments to notify my staff that they would not be able to make it to their scheduled time. We had a waiting list the size of the Superdome and we were usually able to find a patient to move into a vacated slot. It was good for those patients who needed to be seen sooner than I originally could have scheduled them. It was good for business too, because I could only generate revenue when I was actually treating the patient who was physically in front of me.

On the other hand, my staff and I were rendered helpless, sailboats without wind, when a patient called to cancel an appointment one hour before the scheduled office visit. We then did not have any time to contact any other patient to fill that slot and revenue could not be generated. During those times, I would either start working on the piles of charts that had accumulated on my shelves, the charts that I would usually do at night or on weekends, or start calling back patients or doctors that I otherwise would have had to call at the end of the day.

If a patient did not show at the office, we would send a letter requesting him or her to contact us to reschedule the appointment. If anyone was a no show three times, we invoked the "three strikes and you're out (of the practice)" clause. I thought that it was fairly generous of us to give patients each three chances before ejecting them from "our team." Just not to show up was selfish and discourteous to us and other members of community. Some patients, after receiving their ejection letter, called up begging to be reinstated. My staff called me "Dr. Carvel," because many times I was "soft" and said "OK, c'mon back." However, many of those patients who came back no showed again, which then forced us to banish them permanently.

Some of the patients who no showed did not respond to their letters to reschedule and were subsequently put into a category called "lost to follow-up." Some of those patients were never heard from again. That always concerned me. Maybe my staff or I had said something to them that was offensive. (I try to limit the stupid things I say to five per day.) Or maybe I had made errors in their care and they had gone directly to lawyers or other doctors, not questioning me about it first.

Others were heard from when I received phone calls from ER providers, who were evaluating them for conditions that I was treating, but that were now out of control. I was typically worried that these ER providers would think that I had dropped the ball in these persons' care, so I usually started my response, trying to vindicate myself, by saying, "They haven't been seen here in over a year. My notes say they were supposed to come back three months after their last visit, but they no showed and I haven't seen them since. Now, how can I help?"

The last group of "lost to follow-up" patients would not be heard from until their medical conditions had deteriorated so much that they needed to be seen right away. Some, who may have lost all concept of time, would call on Friday afternoons, when my staff and I were typically crawling to the finish line, and ask to be seen urgently or emergently. I usually felt poorly disposed toward such patients. If they had continued to see me on a regular basis, then there might have been something that I could have done to prevent their needing to see me at the end of the day on Friday when everyone else was heading for the weekend.

Continuity of Care is Dead

When I first went into practice, I wanted my patients to know that I was their doctor and that I would be the one responsible for delivering their health care. Although I knew that I could not be available 24/7, I made sure that I not only treated them in the office, but also saw them when they went to the ER or were admitted to the hospital. In that way I could deliver optimal care, because I knew them in both health and sickness. But those days ended years ago. Such continuity of care is dead.

Now there is a series of handoffs from one provider to the next. Some work part-time; some full-time, routinely taking one day off per week. Some are too busy to add patients who become acutely ill, and leave their patients to be seen by someone else, whether in their own offices by mid-level providers or elsewhere, such as an ER or an urgent care center. Some patients are admitted to hospitals and treated by hospitalists, never being seen by their primary care providers, i.e., the physicians responsible for following up and continuing their care after discharge from the hospital. Even the hospitalists work shifts: the 8:00 a.m. to 4:00 p.m. shift, the 4:00 p.m. to midnight shift, and the graveyard shift, midnight to 8:00 a.m., worked by "nocturnalists." Do you think they call it the "graveyard" shift because, by the time the nocturnalists come on, no one knows anything about the patients and that is where the patients end up? Even medical residents learn shift work early in their training with the new residency restriction guidelines. No wonder that patients have come to feel passed around like cheap dates, without anyone taking personal responsibility for their health.

Chapter Sixteen

The Government

"By the People, for the People"

This book is intended to be an account of my experiences as a physician trying to navigate and survive the American health care system. I want to share with you, the reader, the highs and lows of playing in this health care game, so that you may understand why I left my practice at the peak of my career. In previous chapters I used personal stories and vignettes to make my points. This chapter is different. Although its purpose is to delineate our government's role in health care, I have no personal vignettes to share and have had no direct contact with any government official, other than an occasional brief handshake.

That our government's responsibility is to develop policies to serve our population best, including policies on health care, is not open to question. Their decisions and votes have great impact on how clinicians practice medicine and how patients receive health care. No health care policy problems are solvable without some type of government intervention. Thus I feel compelled to comment about our government officials. I must say upfront that I have been disappointed to feel and to live the results of their inaction, their not changing a health care system that rewards a select few while millions more suffer. Maybe the government is the biggest part of the problem.

Ideally, our government officials are voted into office by the people to represent the people. I was not aware that they were voted into office to represent special interest groups, especially in preference to the people. If these officials are to serve the people, then why do so many workers in the health care field feel that special interests trump the citizens of our country when the job is to make health care policy? How do our policy-makers sleep at night, knowing that there are forty-seven million people in America who have no health insurance and millions more who are underinsured, just one bad luck incident away from financial catastrophe? A major cause of personal bankruptcies in 2001 (two million people) was being unable to pay exorbitant medical costs — and half of those people *had* health insurance. According to the Medical Tourism Association <www.medicaltourismassociation.com/>, about half a million Americans opted to travel to other countries in 2006, some even to third-world countries like Costa Rica, for major medical or surgical procedures, because they did not have sufficient health insurance in America. For such patients, to get on planes, travel throughout the world, arrange hotels and food, and pay for health care out of their own pockets was less expensive and less hassle than receiving their medical care in their own homeland, the greatest country in the world.

How could our politicians have allowed the insurance companies to have runaway profits and reserves, to continue to increase their premiums, to refuse health care to those with pre-existing conditions, or to cherry-pick the healthiest patients, all in the name of capitalism and the free market? Do our government officials not believe that health care is a right for all and not just for the healthy or wealthy? Are policy makers not supposed to supply us with basic services like military, police, and fire protection, education, and mail delivery? Does health care not rank as a basic need? How can our country's citizens perform at their jobs and shop — consumerism accounts for two thirds of our GDP — unless they are physically and emotionally well?

How can our government allow the pharmaceutical companies to charge Americans significantly more for medications that can be bought for only a fraction of that cost in other countries? Are individuals in our country so wealthy that we can subsidize the rest of the world's medications? Clearly my patients do not feel that way. Some do not fill or refill expensive prescriptions, preferring instead to use the money for rent, food, or heat. Some only take the pills on occasion, squirreling them away in attempts to make them last longer. Some come in looking for free drug samples to maintain their health. To make matters worse, our government has made it illegal for American residents to fill prescriptions at less cost in other countries, claiming that those medications may be counterfeit or unsafe, even if these medications have been approved by our own FDA. Does the government not recognize what people are trying to say? They are telling the politicians that they are willing to gamble their health by taking possibly counterfeit meds from another country, because the same meds available here, in our own country, are too darn expensive.

Also regarding the cost of medications, could someone please tell me again how and why Medicare Part D turned out to be so bad? It could have been great for our patients and us clinicians alike. We could have prescribed the necessary medications, knowing that our patients could now afford to take them.

Patients who participate in Medicare Part D pay $30 each month to the insurance company, which then covers the cost of their medications up to the first $2510. The patients are then responsible for the next $3600 worth of meds before their insurance kicks in again. This $3600 uncovered cost is called the "donut hole." Who thought of that? What a stupid idea! *Cui bono?* Who benefits?

Is it the insurance companies who collect one and a half billion dollars each year from the monthly $30 premium times 50,000,000 Medicare recipients? Do they get another 180 billion per year if there are 50,000,000 patients in the $3600 "donut hole"? Or is it the pharmaceutical industry that is guaranteed full price for its medications, insofar as Medicare Part D does not allow for any negotiation on drug pricing?

Or is it the lawmakers who — according to data from the *American Journal of Medicine*, April 1, 2004, "Health Care Lobbying in the United States" — were lavished with ninety-six million dollars in 2000 from pharmaceutical and medical supply company lobbyists, which was fifty million dollars more than physicians, nurses, and other health professionals spent combined on trying to promote our agenda? Who are these lawmakers representing anyway? The people who elected them or the insurance and pharmaceutical industries?

Did they think that those patients who could not afford the medications to begin with would all of a sudden have financial windfalls and each be able to pay $3600 out of pocket for the full price? That is why they enrolled in Medicare Part D to begin with. Were they thinking about elderly people on fixed incomes trying to make ends meet each day, each having but one vote at election time? Or were they thinking about themselves and how much money they could all make as they trumpeted Medicare Part D as a fine favor that they were magnanimously doing for our citizens?

Please someone tell me why Medicare did not include the ability to negotiate drug prices with the individual pharmaceutical companies? The government had the leverage and could have negotiated on behalf of our citizens. Our patients were going to purchase a lot of drugs under the Medicare system. The VA, on the other hand, negotiates with these companies and gets deep discounts on their drugs because it purchases in bulk quantities.

What is Good for the Goose is Good for the Gander

The government also makes stringent rules for pharmaceutical companies, limiting the perks that they can give to physicians. I strongly agree with these rules and would consider making them even more stringent. I did not want to have any conflicts of interest when prescribing medications for my patients. I wanted to do what I thought was best for my patients, not what was best for the pharmaceutical industry. Why is it then that, as the government puts limitations on the pharma/physician relationship, there are no limitations on how much money and how many other perks government officials can receive from the pharmaceutical or insurance industry lobbyists?

In addition to the above-mentioned ninety-six million that the pharmaceutical lobbyists spent on government officials in 2000 (and I am sure that they received more than sandwiches or pizza for lunch, pens, and some notepads), the health insurance and managed care company lobbyists spent another thirty-one million to influence U.S. senators and representatives, the White House, and federal agencies that same year. Gary Younge argued in *The Guardian* on January 9, 2006, that "lobbyists have poisoned Washington." Although, since 1995, lobbyists have had to report the organization for which they work and the amount they spend, they have not had to specify how much they spend on entertainment or campaign contributions. Younge quoted Zbigniew Brzezinski's 2002 reaction to lobbyists spending about twenty-five million dollars per politician each year: "A culture has been created in which there is no distinction between what is illegal and what is unethical." From the Clinton to the second Bush administration, the number of lobbyists doubled to 35,000. Since 1998, more than forty per cent of politicians leaving Congress have obtained jobs lobbying their former colleagues. Is there any wonder why so many Americans believe that their legislators are corrupt?

I understand how expensive it is to run a campaign and win an election. The millions of dollars spent on the 2008 presidential campaign by all the candidates were staggering. Mitt Romney alone spent tens of millions of his own money! I accept that to raise that kind of money from individuals is difficult, although Barack Obama was very successful at it in his campaign. I accept that big business has big money and that, without this money, politicians could not easily run for the offices they seek. I also realize that those companies which "invest" in their chosen candidates will want "something" in return for their "contributions." But what I do not agree with, or accept, is making rules and policies that enhance or serve some of the special interest groups, while ignoring or punishing the individuals of our country. After all, it is "the people" who ultimately elect politicians "for the people." Our citizens still matter most. Don't they?

Another bad precedent is when politicians take raises in their own salaries but then cut, or threaten to cut, Medicare reimbursements to physicians. Are we not all in this together? Is there so little money available that we need to cut Medicare expenses? If so, then maybe we should *all* take a financial hit. That would show unity and solidarity. "All for one and one for all, right?" Members of Congress have provided them-

selves, but not us common folk, a retirement plan which pays
them a lifetime pension of full pay, with cost of living increases, even if they only served one term in office — and
100 per cent health care coverage, with no deductibles, prior
approvals, or any limitations at all. Their lifetime plan guaran-
tees these politicians the highest level of health care possible,
and pays their chosen physicians the "usual, customary, and
reasonable fees," not the watered-down fees that the insurance
companies usually pay physicians. What about the rest of us?
Are we chopped liver?

Malpractice premiums are going up and, in certain
states, the cost of that insurance is so prohibitive that some
physicians, like neurosurgeons and obstetrician-gynecologists,
are fleeing those states to set up practice elsewhere, thus
leaving a void in care, especially in rural areas.

Why has there been no tort reform? Physicians are
not perfect. We are human and will make mistakes. Our patients should be compensated if they have suffered from our
errors, but, can the system afford runaway verdicts? Should
there not be some cap on damages? What about the patients
who suffered malpractice but did not have "enough" damages,
i.e., whose cases offered insufficient potential of financial reward, for attorneys to want to take these cases? Should these
patients not have some compensation as well?

From the physicians' point of view, we are being
squeezed from all directions. Reimbursement cuts from
payers necessitates that we see more patients more quickly, to
offset our increasing office expenses. The chances of error
increase as we try to see more patients. This increases our risk
for malpractice. This, in turn, at least in part, increases our
malpractice premiums. Patient outcomes may be suboptimal,
because we physicians do not — or cannot — spend enough
time explaining our patients' conditions, prognoses, and
treatment options to them; or because they cannot afford
their prescribed medications; or, given the many examples of
drug recalls since the 1990s, because they do not trust the
safety of their medications. As a consequence, the patients'
conditions deteriorate, which causes more money to be spent
to treat their worsening health, not to mention their increased

absenteeism or decreased productivity at their jobs. What are physicians, or patients, to do?

Physicians Need a Seat at the Table

In 2007 I attended a lecture given by a prominent policy maker, Judy Feder, who was an advisor to Hillary Clinton in the 1990s when Ms. Clinton made an attempt to modify health care. Feder described some of the problems associated with the contemporary medical environment and outlined proposals to fix these troubles. But she had not included any physicians on any of the committees to reform health care! When I queried her about this during the question-and-answer session, she said she thought that was a good idea. Then why was it not the initial idea?

Years ago my father told me that no one knows a business better than the person who is intricately involved in that business (and my father is never wrong — so he also told me). Then who knows how to deliver health care best, a policy maker or a physician? What is their training in the field of medicine? We are the ones who have to feel good about the rules that govern us, so why not have us more intimately involved in the process? Better representation on government committees would allow us to give additional insight and understanding to the complex problems of maintaining our nation's health and treating our population's diseases.

Why would our politicians and policy makers think that they could solve the health care system without physicians' input? At no time have I heard any candidate from either the Republican or Democratic side say, "I discussed these issues with representatives from the various medical societies, organizations, boards, and the surgeon general, and this is what we think would be best to serve the people of our country." There was not one physician on Clinton's team in the 1990s. Are we just pawns in their game? When they say jump, are we supposed to ask, "How high?" Let us pull up a chair at the table.

Chapter Seventeen

Back to Clinical Medicine

Too Young to Retire

"But, you're too young to retire," my mother said to me in her strong Brooklyn accent when I told her that I was leaving the practice of medicine with the closing of the DEC. I kidded her that there is something called "doctor years" (a term I made up on the spot) which is analogous to "dog years." The thought is that every year a dog lives equals seven human years. As a medical student, resident, and doctor, I worked "like a dog" somewhere between sixty and 120 hours per week for over twenty-five years, which is equal to well over forty years of work for the typical non-medical American who works forty hours a week. I just happened to have worked those forty years in twenty-five "doctor years."

I certainly am not leaving medicine and retiring. How could I? I do not golf, fish, or whittle, and I loathe puttering around the house. And my mother is right (no surprise): I am too young and still too ambitious and motivated to retire.

My Idealism Lives On

During my months out of medical practice I had countless people say to me, "You look so relaxed." I did not know whether to say "Thank you" or to feel bad that I had looked so terribly stressed when I had been trying to serve my community and alleviate its medical problems. But I know, without question, that my balding and graying has stabilized, I have lost several pounds, and my general "aggravation level" has come way down.

I got into the routine over the years, before going to sleep each night, of reminiscing about the day just passed and deciding whether it was "perfect." That would be a day in which everything went flawlessly, from the mundane, like all the lights being green on the way to work, to the extreme, like being able to make an accurate diagnosis for a patient with a complicated medical history. All in all, prior to my last day in clinical practice, I counted about seven perfect days in that practice from 1991 to 2007. In the next seven months after being out of practice, I believe I had about six months' worth of perfect days.

I have noticed that my use of expletive has gone way down from several "motherf---ers" a day to about one a month. I never set my alarm clock. I do not wear a watch. I sleep eight to nine hours each night, exercise for at least one hour each day, and thus far have achieved the goals that I set for myself after I left practice: not doing the same thing two days in a row, not working more than ten hours in a day, and not taking less than thirty minutes to eat lunch. Yet, each morning when I opened my eyes, I felt a significant void. I was not contributing to my community, nor was I doing what I was trained to do, helping people with their medical conditions. Frankly, aside from all the non-clinical nonsense, that was what I had enjoyed doing.

"Mirror, mirror on the wall, what was it that inspired me to become a doctor anyway?" I said to myself in the mirror each morning after leaving practice. Writing this book has forced me to be introspective, to reassess in midlife, and to consider the many aspects of being and wanting to be a doctor. It has also forced me to remember who and where I was when I decided to become one. What was I looking for that made me want to spend the time, energy, and money to go to medical school, persevere, and survive training, and work endless hours under substantial stress while in practice. Would it be possible, once I find those answers, to rekindle my enthusiasm and zest to want to return to clinical medicine?

I remember very clearly and distinctly that I wanted to be a doctor to serve those who needed help, while testing myself mentally and physically, pushing myself to the "max," to do something I that was not sure I could do. I looked forward to learning about and using all the incredible advances in medical science, better to serve my patients, and the opportunity to discuss those advances and nuances with other physicians. I also hoped that I would one day become proficient enough with knowledge, wisdom, and experiences to be able to teach other doctors who were trying to climb the medical ladder. *Doctor* in Latin means "leader" or "teacher," from the infinitive *docere*, which means "to lead" or "to teach."

After being in practice for over sixteen years, I also discovered that, although I like to work hard and push myself to my limits, I also know that life is short and being able to have balance between work and non-work, with time to develop personal relationships and pursue life's other wonderments, is also important. I picture lying on my deathbed one day, I hope still at home and with my bladder and bowels still under my control. Would I be wishing that I had spent more time at work, not pursuing outside experiences and developing relationships, or would I regret that I had not had balance in life?

I also realized that being in clinical practice is basically a dead-end — (I hesitate to use the words "clinical practice" and "dead" in the same sentence) — job with no room for advancement. The best I could hope for would be to continue more of the same, i.e., continue only to see patients, all day, every day, "line 'em up, knock 'em down."

I yearned for an improved medical record system to improve the care of my patients: a system that could not only maintain records from years ago, but could also give me immediate access to medical care that a patient of mine had just received, whether notes from previous doctors, labs, or even the actual x-rays — even if the care had been given at a different institution or another medical office. No longer would my staff have to sit endlessly on the phone. No longer would we have to rely on the patient's memory to learn what had actually been done.

Because I despise living under the constant threat of malpractice litigation, is there a place where I could deliver my best possible care, understanding that medicine is far from a perfect science and that bad outcomes are inevitable, despite yeoman's efforts, and where I would not be distracted that a lawsuit might be only the next patient away?

So, is there a place where idealistic clinicians, like me, can practice medicine and have many of their other needs met? The answer, miraculously, is "yes," and it is at the place with "The Best Care Anywhere."

Serving Those Who Served

"The Best Care Anywhere" was the title of an article written by Phillip Longman for the January/February 2005 *Washington Monthly* that described the ascent of the VA hospital system. In 2007 PoliPoint Press published his book, *Best Care Anywhere: Why VA Health Care is Better Than Yours.* Years ago, the reputation of the VA hospitals was soiled by poor medical care and decaying facilities. However, over the last several years the VA has upgraded its facilities, especially in Syracuse. Our VA <www.syracuse.va.gov/> has been ranked number one in the country for several measures of quality of care, patient access, and patient satisfaction, among VAs of similar size. Many vibrant physicians who still "have gas in the tank" and want to practice "good" medicine, without the non-clinical aggravations of being in private practice, have gravitated to the VA to work, and not just to "live out" the remainder of their careers, too burned out to deliver the quality of care our military heroes deserve, getting a paycheck, and collecting benefits.

I "enlisted" at the Syracuse Veterans Administration Medical Center and started working there on June 23, 2008, as a hospitalist, treating veterans in the hospital for their acute illnesses. "Why work at the VA?" I've been asked many times. Let me give you my top ten reasons:

First and foremost, I have been deeply moved by the incredibly brave men and women who have served in our military over the generations, most recently in Iraq and Afghanistan, and have returned injured, either physically or mentally. Maybe I am so moved because I have children the same age as those who are serving (it could have been one of my kids coming home mutilated), or maybe because of the graphic scenes in movies like *Saving Private Ryan*, or maybe because of the guilt that I harbor within me that I never served in my country's military. Maybe it is some combination of these, but, in any case, I feel compelled to serve those who have served. It is my way of giving back to those who have given to us what some of us may take for granted, our freedom.

Second, it is a wonderful chance to be around other physicians, to share medical knowledge and nuances, and to work together as a team to give the patients optimal care. While I was in private practice, I basically had my head down, focused on treating problem after problem, using my knowledge and wits. There were only limited discussions and sharing of ideas with other doctors during the course of each day, something I had enjoyed when I was in training.

Third, because the VA is a teaching hospital associated with Upstate Medical University, across the street, medical students and doctors in training come through the VA during their different rotations. For me, therefore, it is a wonderful opportunity to relearn some of the general medicine that I used to love to know and to teach residents, interns, and medical students. I still feel at the top of my game, with a thirst and desire to learn more myself, to help the patients even more. I know that I do not know everything. I wish I did; life would be so much easier.

Fourth, the VA medical record system is the best in the country, because all the VAs are connected electronically, which helps the VA providers to keep track of veterans' medical conditions, labs, x-rays, and consultations. This not only improves the continuity of care, but also reduces costs, medical errors, and duplication of services, something that non-VA EMR services have not even come close to promoting. Imagine that a veteran could be seen in a VA ER in Texas yesterday and the records would be available to me in Syracuse today when he shows up in our ER. No nurse has to sit on the phone making phone calls trying to find out what the patient's problems and solutions were when he was seen the day before, and all his records, dating back thirty years, are available in the data bank.

Fifth, there could be opportunities to do more for the advance of medicine than just patient care, such as administrative work, or even formulating protocols that could be used nationwide. For example, the protocols that the chief of the Syracuse VA ER wrote for treating ER patients are now used across the country. I may be able to write protocols for treating diabetics in the hospital to reduce morbidity, mortality, and length of stay, or for helping in end-of-life care.

Sixth, there is flexibility and the option for me to transfer to another VA hospital in another part of the country, without losing any financial benefits, if my wife and I were ever to tire of the seemingly endless winters in Central New York.

Seventh, as a hospitalist, I would work two sixty-hour weeks, fourteen days in a row then have a week off. When we added in vacation time and federal holidays, I would work sixty hours per week, twenty-eight and a half weeks per year, and even be given sick days if I needed them. When I was in private-sector practice, I worked sixty-hour weeks about forty-eight weeks per year and took only one sick day in over sixteen years. Imagine, a balance between contributing to my community and still having time to see my family and to pursue interests outside the field of medicine! I would not even have to schlep bags of patients' papers home at night or sit in right field doing paperwork while still trying to enjoy my kid's baseball game.

Eighth, I do not have to concern myself with whether the patients have Medicare, Medicaid, private insurance, or no insurance, or how they are going to pay me. There is only one set of rules to deal with and to remember. I do not have to worry about different criteria from different insurance companies, or who will or will not cover which test, nor will I concern myself with preauthorizations, precertifications, letters of denial for care, nor letters of rejection for services.

Also, the personal financial benefits are competitive. As the VA recruiter said to me during the recruitment process, I may not become the wealthiest doctor in the world — as if that was ever important to me — but my salary would never go down, something I certainly could not say when I was in fee-for-service practice. Plus, there are all the federal retirement and insurance benefits. Like a professional athlete, I even received a signing bonus! Imagine, they gave me money just for coming to a place that I wanted to come to anyway! Remember, I enlisted in the VA system, I was not drafted.

Ninth, I would not have to worry about staff showing up or not showing up. I had great admiration and respect for my staff when I was in non-government practice, but there was no one to "pull off the bench" or "bring out of the bullpen" if someone did not show up on a particular day. On those days, those that did show up either did more work or the work just did not get done. At the VA, it is the hospital administration's responsibility to make sure that there is a sufficient number of nurses and ancillary workers available for each shift on each day to make sure that the hospital runs smoothly and that the patients are well cared for.

Tenth, if patients ever felt like they had malpractice done against them, they would not be able to sue any individual provider, but rather, they would have to sue the federal government, typically under the Federal Tort Claims Act of 1946. This does not mean that providers should not continue to be ultradiligent with their patients, treating them as "our own," but just takes away the looming threat — and the aggravation that goes along with it — that at any time we could be individually named in a malpractice suit.

I have no delusions that working at the VA will be perfect; no place is. But, compared with practicing medicine in the "real world," it has so far been a breath of fresh air. At least I have to give it a chance to be the holy grail that I have been seeking. Thus, if there is any place where I can go and be the doctor that I have dreamed of being, then the VA may be the best place for me, anywhere.

Chapter Eighteen

Solutions

It Does Not Have to Be This Way

The old riddle goes, how many psychiatrists does it take to change a light bulb? One, but the light bulb has to want to change. I believe that this is the major problem with reforming the American health care system in the early twenty-first century: There is no motivation or incentive for the people who are benefiting or profiting the most from it to *want* to change. Maybe they do not perceive a problem. Maybe they are blind to the inequities. Or maybe they just do not care about the unfairness that exists and maybe they say, "Hooray for me and to hell with you." While they put up obstacles against change, and "spin" their own importance in maintaining the health care system as it is, many people in our nation are suffering and even dying because of it. What is most upsetting to me, as a guy caught in the middle, is that it just does not have to be this way. It could all be so much better.

Some have said that, if anyone started from scratch, they would not have concocted the American health care system. Why would anyone who truly cared about the physical and emotional health of our citizens — the people who build our cities, farm our fields, and teach our children — put together a system where a select few, including the insurance and pharmaceutical companies, malpractice attorneys, and even some physicians, make (take?) obscene amounts of money from the system while many others, our forty-seven million people in America, go without health care? Are these forty-seven million uninsured, and many others who are partially or inadequately insured, not worthy of health care? We spend more money per capita than any other country on health care. There are a few who "have" and too many who "have not." Despite all this money, over two trillion dollars per year, the WHO still ranked our health care performance thirty-seventh in the world in 2000. The situation has not improved.

Since I started seeing patients as a third-year medical student in 1983, I have witnessed first-hand the agonizing decisions that many people or their family members have had to make trying to decide if they should eat, pay the heating bill, see the doctor, or buy the prescribed medicine. People have to stay at dissatisfying jobs or risk changing employment and losing their health insurance, because they might have "preexisting conditions." I have seen two of my patients die because *they* had to decide whether *they* were sick enough to go to the ER and spend that money, or well enough to wait it out and hope that they would just miraculously get better. Putting such decisions, whether to see medical providers or not, into the hands of untrained, ordinary people is extremely dangerous. I told my patients that one of the best ways to use a clinician's expertise is when they were not sure if their medical concerns were significant or not. If you are not sure, then call.

In only about twenty years I have seen the health insurance industry dramatically augment their financial reservoirs, raise our patients' premiums, increase their intrusion into our practices, and adversely affect our medical decision-making, all while reaping more profit than ever. What do our patients get in return? Shorter office visits, longer waits to be seen, skepticism of their physicians' intentions — the "they're-just-trying-to-make-money-off-me" attitude — and general dissatisfaction with being patients. I believe that most doctors could be interested in helping to manage medical costs. But it is repugnant, at least to me, that the money thus saved goes into the insurance companies' own pockets. More dollars in the system has certainly not translated into better care.

Many of us physicians are pushed, as a consequence of lower reimbursements and rising expenses, to work longer days, to see more patients each day, and to see them more quickly, lest we "go out of practice" for "business reasons," like the DEC. This is not how we were taught in medical school. It is not good for the patients nor is it good for the providers. It is dangerous! The chance for mistakes is greater when clinicians have to make their best decisions after less time with patients to gather information and communicate their thoughts back to them. Moreover, patients are more apt to sue when they and their clinicians have not established sufficient rapport and when they feel like their physicians did not take enough time with them. Malpractice premiums are increasing, despite stability in jury awards and malpractice settlements. Some physicians' malpractice premium burdens are so great that they have moved away from certain cities and counties, leaving those citizens without necessary medical services, such as neurosurgery and obstetrics.

Many medical students leave four years of undergraduate and four years of medical school with debt of over $100,000. Given the large disparity in the pay of different kinds of physicians, many medical school graduates choose to practice higher-paying medical and surgical specialties, which leaves a significant shortage of primary care physicians, such as family practitioners, internists, pediatricians, and even psychiatrists and endocrinologists. This comes at a time when our population is becoming more obese, older, and more depressed. Many insured people already have only limited access to medical care, given the scarcity of primary care providers. Likely this will just get worse, especially if universal health care is mandated and a tsunami of forty-seven million more people in America go looking for primary care providers, or even endocrinologists.

We have seen the pharmaceutical industry attain and maintain profitability greater than any other industry in the world. We have witnessed pharmaceutical companies come out with expensive new medications and unneeded "me-too" drugs, and profit handsomely from them. Meanwhile, many of my patients did not or could not fill or refill the prescriptions I gave them, but squirreled away the medications that they had, trying to save them like precious metals; or they came to my office to beg for samples, hoping to stay on their meds to stay healthy and well, but knowing that they could not afford these meds.

What was equally distressing to me, after all my years of training and practicing medicine, was that I felt as if I had become just a conduit, a tool, for insurance and pharmaceutical companies to make their profits. I also felt like I was a target for malpractice attorneys and a pawn of government officials, who seemed to worry more about raising money from special interests than about serving our citizens. Physicians are very unhappy with our system. Many feel burned out. Recall that the 2007 ACPE survey, cited above in Chapter Two, claimed that sixty per cent had already considered leaving practice prematurely, given the American health care environment.

Patients have also contributed to our health care problems. Over thirty per cent of our adults and almost twenty per cent of our children are either overweight or frankly obese, and these percentages are increasing annually. It is clear that medical consequences associated with weight, like diabetes, hypertension, hyperlipidemia, vascular disease, arthritis, sleep apnea, and depression — just to name a few — put an extra financial burden on our health care system. Many patients still smoke, increasing their risk for not only vascular disease but also emphysema, bronchitis, and lung cancer. Other patients, even those with insurance, do not have up-to-date vaccinations, do not go for routine checkups, or do not obtain the recommended screening tests, like mammograms, prostate exams, or colorectal exams. Preventing disease or diagnosing it earlier can improve patient outcomes and in the end will cost the system less. What about end-of-life care? Per capita we spend more health care money on people in their last year of life than in their previous years combined. How do we remain ethical and moral without breaking the health care bank?

I am certain that our health care system could be so much better if everyone were willing to give up something to make the system best for most. But I understand that instituting change can be very difficult.

At a dinner party of about sixteen people I became engaged in a passionate discussion about the health care system. Many at the table were professionals who had studied and worked extremely hard to achieve their successes. They understood the plight of the uninsured and inadequately insured and the drawbacks of the American system, but many at the table were satisfied with their current, albeit expensive, insurance plans and the health care that they and their families were receiving. They were very skeptical of change. They seemed to suspect that any new system would be worse for them —

more expensive, with reduced access and administrative incompetence, for example. When I proposed alternative plans to the current system, I was met with considerable resistance. Attempts to give any details were quickly rejected.

Despite some people's reservations about a change from the prevailing system, I do believe that the status quo must go, being too sick to survive. Resuscitating the health care system will take more than a Band-Aid, Steri-Strip, splint, or cast. We will not be able to fix it just by taking out its gallbladder or appendix and hoping that the rest of the system will get better. All the elements are interwoven and connected. Like the knee bone is connected to the thigh bone and the thigh bone is connected to the hip bone, so is the government connected to the type of payer, the pharmaceutical companies, and tort reform. The payers, pharma, and malpractice attorneys are connected to the physicians and the physicians are connected to the patients, who are also connected to payers, pharma, and at times, malpractice attorneys. Failing to address everything that is broken will not maximally or even satisfactorily fix anything that is broken. We need a "full court press," a total systems change to repair this failing system. How many people will it take to change the system? Everyone, but the system has to want to change.

My Wish List

In the preceding chapters I have tried to outline the problems of the health care system from my vantage point as a physician in the trenches. I used vignettes and stories to highlight issues. I feel certain that there can be a better system, which would be best for most. Frankly it is not important to me who comes up with the best idea to solve our health care ills, just as long as improvements come about. As I told my patients, "I don't care who gets you better as long as you get better." Let's put all the egos away.

I admit to idealism, but as far as I am concerned the only things that cannot be changed are the heavenly bodies, the tides, and Mother Nature. That said, from a practical standpoint, we may need to take baby steps until the final plan is in place.

There are very many scholarly, articulate people who have studied health care from a variety of angles and have written books and other publications outlining and defending their ideas and positions. I am not in their league. I only know that there is too much pain and suffering in the system and I wish it could be better. Therefore, why not form a non-partisan commission and put all the "P's" in one "pod"? Sequester representatives of the Politicians, Policy makers, Pundits, Physicians, Payers, Patients, Plaintiffs' attorneys, and Pharmaceutical companies all in a room, and do not let them out until they configure a plan that is best for most, understanding that everyone will have to give up something and that no one will get everything.

The following is my wish list. I know that a genie coming out of a bottle usually grants just three wishes, but I have taken the liberty of asking for "lucky thirteen." I hope that when the final horn has sounded and the system has been decided upon, some of what is on my list will be included:

1. Give everyone access to affordable health care.
2. Keep things simple for patients, providers, and the administrators of the system.
3. Eliminate any potential for conflict of interest. Find and prosecute anyone trying to defraud the system.
4. Offer lower-priced medications to help patients maintain adherence with their treatment plans.
5. Enforce less disparity in physician incomes to attract more physicians to primary care.
6. Create strong incentives for patients to seek preventive care and pursue healthier lifestyles.
7. Institute tort reform.
8. Improve FDA oversight to ensure that medications are as safe as possible.
9. Use independent research companies to study new medications.
10. Train enough clinicians and nurses, so that they can spend more time with their patients.
11. Support more evidenced-based research and institute cost-effective guidelines for clinicians to follow.
12. Reduce paperwork by facilitating better communication

among physicians, and between physicians and patients, with a universal EMR system or with patients maintaining their own records on computer chips or smart cards that would be updated after each visit.
13. Provide end-of-life care that is compassionate, ethical, moral, and cost-effective.

I do not know if our politicians have the will or the courage to initiate change or if our medical societies have the desire or the clout to instigate reforms. Maybe it will take a grass roots movement of the people to prompt change or a "million person march" on Washington.

I told my wife, when I left my practice and wanted to write a book about my experiences as an American physician at the beginning of the twenty-first century, that I hoped for five miracles:

The first miracle would be that I could write a book. The last non-scientific paper that I recall writing was in 1978, when I was a junior in college, and I received a B minus. My typing skills are weak and I knew that writing a book would be analogous to shoveling snow from my driveway with a spoon.

The second would be that my book would get published.

The third would be that someone would read it. If you are reading this book now, then I have already achieved my first three miracles.

The fourth would be that the book would become widely popular and, just for the fun of it, I would go on *The Daily Show* and, of course, *Oprah*. If a movie were ever made of it, who would be better to play me than ... ?

The last miracle, which was far and away my main objective, would be to give further insight into the problems of the American health care system at the beginning of this century from a physician's point of view. I left my practice to speak out and to give examples about the problems of this system, with hopes that it could be so much better. I hope my voice has been heard. If anything constructive comes from this book, I would then feel that my loss of income and the time away from my patients was well worth it.